T0326319

Curbside Consultation in Glaucoma

49 Clinical Questions

Second UPDATED Edition

CURBSIDE CONSULTATION IN OPHTHALMOLOGY
SERIES

SERIES EDITOR, DAVID F. CHANG, MD

Second
UPDATED
Edition

Curbside Consultation in Glaucoma

49 Clinical Questions

Editor
Steven J. Gedde, MD
Bascom Palmer Eye Institute
Miami, Florida

Associate Editors
Dale K. Heuer, MD
Richard A. Lewis, MD
Joseph F. Panarelli, MD

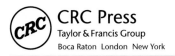

CRC Press
Taylor & Francis Group
Boca Raton London New York

CRC Press is an imprint of the
Taylor & Francis Group, an **informa** business

First Published in 2015 by SLACK Incorporated

Published 2024 by CRC Press
2385 NW Executive Center Drive, Suite 320, Boca Raton FL 33431

and by CRC Press
4 Park Square, Milton Park, Abingdon, Oxon, OX14 4RN

CRC Press is an imprint of Taylor & Francis Group, an informa business

Although Dr. Heuer and Dr. Gedde serve as American Board of Ophthalmology (ABO) board director and examiner, respectively, and Dr. Gedde is an American Academy of Ophthalmology Ophthalmic Knowledge Assessment Program (OKAP) committee member, this work and its content shall not be marketed or construed as ABO or OKAP preparatory material. Furthermore, the views expressed herein do not necessarily reflect those of any organization listed above.

Library of Congress Cataloging-in-Publication Data

Curbside consultation in glaucoma : 49 clinical questions / editor, Steven J. Gedde. — Second edition.
  p. ; cm. — (Curbside consultation in ophthalmology series)
  Includes bibliographical references and index.
  ISBN 978-1-61711-639-1 (paperback : alk. paper)
  I. Gedde, Steven J., editor.   II. Series: Curbside consultation in ophthalmology series.
  [DNLM: 1. Glaucoma—diagnosis.   2. Glaucoma—therapy. WW 290]
  RE871
  617.7'41—dc23

                                                                    2014036751

ISBN: 9781617116391 (pbk)
ISBN: 9781003523543 (ebk)

DOI: 10.1201/9781003523543

Dedication

We dedicate this book to our families for bringing balance to our lives, to our mentors for sharing their wisdom with us, and to our patients for showing us how to persevere with a chronic disease.

Contents

Acknowledgments

We would like to acknowledge David Chang for his creativity in developing the *Curbside Consultation* series. We thank all authors for sharing their practical wisdom. We are grateful to the residents and clinicians who provided feedback to guide the content of this book. Finally, we appreciate all of the hard work from the team at SLACK, including Tony Schiavo, Erika Gonzalez, Katherine Rola, April Billick, Michelle Gatt, Lyndee Stalter, and John Bond.

About the Editor

Steven J. Gedde, MD is Professor of Ophthalmology and Vice Chairman of Education at the Bascom Palmer Eye Institute. He received his medical degree from Vanderbilt University School of Medicine. Dr Gedde completed his residency training in ophthalmology at Wills Eye Hospital, where he also served as Chief Resident. His clinical glaucoma fellowship was done at the Bascom Palmer Eye Institute.

Dr. Gedde has lectured nationally and internationally. He has authored or coauthored more than 250 articles, book chapters, and abstracts. He serves on the Editorial Boards for *Ophthalmology, Journal of Academic Ophthalmology, EyeNet, Ocular Surgery News, Ophthalmology Management,* and *EyeWorld*. Dr. Gedde has been listed among *Best Doctors in America* since 2005, and he received the American Academy of Ophthalmology Achievement Award in 2006 and Senior Achievement Award in 2012. He has served as the Residency Program Director at the Bascom Palmer Eye Institute since 1999, and he was selected as the Excellence in Health Care Educator of the Year in 2009. Dr. Gedde is also a study chairman for the Tube Versus Trabeculectomy (TVT) Study and Primary Tube Versus Trabeculectomy (PTVT) Study, multicenter randomized clinical trials comparing tube shunt surgery with trabeculectomy.

About the Associate Editors

Dale K. Heuer, MD received his undergraduate and medical degrees from Northwestern University. He completed his ophthalmology residency at the Medical College of Wisconsin and a two year National Research Service Award-funded glaucoma fellowship at the Bascom Palmer Eye Institute, University of Miami School of Medicine. He served on the full-time faculty of the University of Florida College of Medicine (1984–1986) and University of Southern California School of Medicine (1986–1997). Since 1997, Dr. Heuer has been professor and chairman of Ophthalmology at the Medical College of Wisconsin, where he also serves as the director of the Froedtert and the Medical College of Wisconsin Eye Institute.

He has published extensively on the use of conventional filtering procedures with wound-healing modulation and aqueous shunting procedures for the management of glaucomas with poor surgical prognoses. Dr. Heuer has participated in several glaucoma clinical trials, including the Fluorouracil Filtering Surgery Study, the Collaborative Normal-Tension Glaucoma Study, and the Collaborative Initial Glaucoma Study. He was also one of the three vice chairs of the National Eye Institute-sponsored Ocular Hypertension Treatment Study.

Dr. Heuer currently serves in the following capacities: Board director for the American Board of Ophthalmology; co-chair of the Tube Versus Trabeculectomy Study; member of the Safety & Data Monitoring Committees of the Ahmed-Baerveldt Comparison Study, Primary Tube versus Trabeculectomy Study, and Ghana Primary Tube versus Trabeculectomy Study; and consulting member of the U.S. Food & Drug Administration's Ophthalmic Device Panel. He was the founding board chair and is a current board member for Friends for Health in Haiti.

Richard A. Lewis, MD is the former director of glaucoma at the University of California, Davis. In addition to his busy clinical practice located in Sacramento, California, Dr. Lewis is actively involved in clinical research in national and international trials in anterior segment disease and glaucoma therapy. He is the current President of the American Society of Cataract and Refractive Surgery (2014–2015) and past president of the American Glaucoma Society (2000–2002). Dr. Lewis is the medical Editor Emeritus of *Glaucoma Today* and on the editorial board of the *Journal of Cataract and Refractive Surgery, Journal of Glaucoma, Video Journal of Ophthalmology,* and *Ocular Surgery News.* He is cofounder of Sacramento's Capital City Surgery Center (2003).

Dr. Lewis attended the University of California, Berkeley as an undergraduate and received his doctorate in medicine from Northwestern University Medical School in Chicago in 1978. His ophthalmology training included a residency at the Department of Ophthalmology at the University of California, Davis, and a fellowship in glaucoma at the University Of Iowa Department Of Ophthalmology in Iowa City (1982-83). He is a Diplomat of the American Board of Ophthalmology and the National Board of Medical Examiners.

Dr. Lewis has published over eighty articles and book chapters focusing on glaucoma, ophthalmic surgery, and ophthalmic pharmacology. He teaches and lectures extensively on glaucoma and cataract surgery. He has received the American Academy of Ophthalmology Honor and Senior Honor as well as the Secretariat and Life Achievement Awards for his contributions in teaching and leadership and for initiating the AAO Subspecialty Day meeting.

A native of San Francisco, Dr. Lewis lives in Sacramento with his wife; the couple has two grown children.

Joseph F. Panarelli, MD is an assistant professor of ophthalmology at the New York Eye and Ear Infirmary of Mount Sinai, where he specializes in the treatment of glaucoma. Dr. Panarelli received his medical degree from the Georgetown University School of Medicine. He then completed his ophthalmology residency at the New York Eye and Ear Infirmary and served as chief resident during his final year of training. He was awarded the William and Judith Turner Award for excellence in ophthalmologic training. He completed a fellowship in glaucoma at the Bascom Palmer Eye Institute and subsequently joined the faculty there. He later transitioned back to the New York Eye and Ear Infirmary of Mount Sinai, where he was appointed the Associate Residency Program Director.

Dr. Panarelli has published multiple original articles and book chapters, and he has presented his research at national and international conferences. He is an investigator for several studies pertaining to the surgical management of glaucoma and is currently studying the effects of transient intraocular pressure elevation on the optic nerve with support from the Empire Clinical Research Investigator Program.

Contributing Authors

Iqbal Ike K. Ahmed, MD, FRCSC (Question 47)
Trillium Health Partners, GoEyeCare
University of Toronto,
Oakville, Ontario, Canada

R. Rand Allingham, MD (Question 17)
Richard and Kit Barkhouser Professor of
  Ophthalmology
Director, Glaucoma Service
Duke University Eye Center
Durham, North Carolina

Douglas R. Anderson, MD, FARVO (Question 3)
Professor *Emeritus* of Ophthalmology
Bascom Palmer Eye Institute
University of Miami School of
  Medicine
Douglas R. Anderson Distinguished Chair in
  Ophthalmology
Miami, Florida

Husam Ansari, MD, PhD (Question 20)
Ophthalmic Consultants of Boston
Boston, Massachusetts

Ahmad A. Aref, MD (Question 41)
Illinois Eye and Ear Infirmary
University of Illinois College of Medicine
Chicago, Illinois

Michael Banitt, MD (Question 14)
University of Miami Miller School of
  Medicine
Miami, Florida

Andrew J. Barkmeier, MD (Question 18)
Assistant Professor, Department of
  Ophthalmology
Mayo Clinic
Rochester, Minnesota

*Keith Barton, MD, FRCP, FRCS
  (Question 39)*
Moorfields Eye Hospital
London, England

Dana M. Blumberg, MD, MPH (Question 11)
Assistant Professor of Ophthalmology
Columbia University
Department of Ophthalmology
Harkness Eye Institute
New York, New York

James D. Brandt, MD (Question 12)
Professor of Ophthalmology and Vision Science
Director, Glaucoma Service
UC Davis Eye Center
Sacramento, California

Adam C. Breunig, MD (Question 8)
Chicago Glaucoma Consultants
Rush University Medical Center
Chicago, Illinois

Donald L. Budenz, MD, MPH (Question 44)
Department of Ophthalmology
Kittner Family Distinguished Professor and
  Chair
University of North Carolina
Chapel Hill, North Carolina

Joseph Caprioli, MD (Question 10)
Professor of Ophthalmology
David May II Chair in Ophthalmology
UCLA David Geffen School of Medicine
Chief, Glaucoma Division, UCLA Stein Eye
Los Angeles, California

Ta Chen Peter Chang, MD (Question 23)
Assistant Professor of Ophthalmology
University of Miami Miller School of Medicine
Bascom Palmer Eye Institute
Miami, Florida

Philip P. Chen, MD (Question 1)
Professor and Grace E. Hill Chair
Department of Ophthalmology
Chief of Ophthalmology
University of Washington Medicine Eye
  Institute
Seattle, Washington

E. Randy Craven, MD, FACS (Question 4)
Chief of Glaucoma
King Khaled Eye Specialist Hospital
Riyadh, Saudi Arabia
Associate Professor
Wilmer Eye Institute
Johns Hopkins University
Baltimore, Maryland

David L. Cute, DO (Question 29)
Walter Reed National Military Medical
    Center
Bethesda, Maryland

Igor Estrovich, MD (Question 45)
Devers Eye Institute
Portland, Oregon

Francisco Fantes, MD (Question 29)
Deceased

Ronald L. Fellman, MD (Question 40)
Attending Surgeon and Clinician
Glaucoma Associates of Texas
Associate Clinical Professor Emeritus
Department of Ophthalmology
University of Texas Southwestern Medical
    Center
Dallas, Texas

John H. Fingert, MD, PhD (Question 16)
Department of Ophthalmology and Visual
    Sciences
Carver College of Medicine
University of Iowa
Glaucoma Research Center
Wynn Institute of Vision
    Research
Iowa City, Iowa

*David Fleischman, MD, MS
    (Question 17)*
Fellow, Duke University Eye
    Center
Durham, North Carolina

Brian A. Francis, MD, MS (Question 35)
Professor of Ophthalmology
David Geffen School of Medicine
University of California
Los Angeles, California

David S. Greenfield, MD (Question 15)
Professor of Ophthalmology
Bascom Palmer Eye Institute
University of Miami Miller School of
    Medicine
Miami, Florida

*Davinder S. Grover, MD, MPH
    (Questions 26, 40)*
Attending Clinician and Surgeon
Glaucoma Associates of Texas
Clinical Assistant Professor
University of Texas, Southwestern Medical
    School
Dallas, Texas

Gregg A. Heatley, MD (Question 21)
University of Wisconsin
Department of Ophthalmology and Visual
    Sciences
Madison, Wisconsin

Wendy W. Huang, MD (Question 30)
New York Eye and Ear Infirmary of Mount
    Sinai
New York, New York

Annisa L. Jamil, MD (Question 22)
Glaucoma Consultants North West
Seattle, Washington

Anna K. Junk, MD (Question 19)
Associate Professor of Ophthalmology
Bascom Palmer Eye Institute
University of Miami Miller School of
    Medicine
Director of Glaucoma Service
Miami Veterans Affairs Healthcare System
Miami, Florida

Malik Y. Kahook, MD (Question 48)
Department of Ophthalmology
The Slater Family Endowed Chair and
    Professor of Ophthalmology
University of Colorado School of
    Medicine
Aurora, Colorado

Dima Kalache, MD, CM (Question 49)
McGill University Health Center
Department of Ophthalmology
Montreal, Canada

Anne Ko, MD (Question 14)
University of Miami Miller School of
    Medicine
Miami, Florida

Dennis Lam, MD, FRCOphth (Question 46)
State Key Laboratory of Ophthalmology
Sun Yat-Sen University
Hong Kong, China

Paul P. Lee, MD, JD (Question 11)
F. Bruce Fralick Professor and Chair
    of Ophthalmology and Visual
    Sciences
University of Michigan
Director, W.K. Kellogg Eye Center
Ann Arbor, Michigan

Richard K. Lee, MD, PhD (Question 33)
Associate Professor of Ophthalmology
Bascom Palmer Eye Institute
University of Miami Miller School of
    Medicine
Miami, Florida

*Christopher Leung, MD, MSc, BMedSc, MB,
    ChB (Question 7)*
Department of Ophthalmology and Visual
    Sciences
The Chinese University of Hong Kong
Hong Kong, China

Enne Liang, PhD (Question 46)
Dennis Lam and Partners Eye
    Center
Hong Kong, China

Jeffrey M. Liebmann, MD (Question 37)
Department of Ophthalmology
New York University School of
    Medicine
New York, New York

John T. Lind, MD, MS (Question 18)
Assistant Professor, Department of
    Ophthalmology and Visual
    Sciences
Washington University
Saint Louis, Missouri

Jane Loman, MD (Question 10)
Eye Physicians of East Bay
Oakland, California

Steven L. Mansberger, MD, MPH (Question 45)
Devers Eye Institute
Portland, Oregon

Rashmi G. Mathew, FRCOphth (Question 39)
Moorfields Eye Hospital
London, England

Hylton R. Mayer, MD (Question 28)
Eye Doctors of Washington
Chevy Chase, Maryland

Felipe A. Medeiros, MD, PhD (Question 6)
Ben and Wanda Hildyard Chair for Diseases
    of the Eye
Professor of Ophthalmology
University of California San Diego
San Diego, California

Richard P. Mills, MD, MPH (Question 22)
Glaucoma Consultants North West
Seattle, Washington

Silvia Orengo-Nania, MD (Question 34)
Professor, Department of Ophthalmology
Baylor College of Medicine
Eye Care Line Executive
Michael E. DeBakey VAMC
Houston, Texas

Sung Chul Park, MD (Question 24)
Assistant Professor of Ophthalmology
Manhattan Eye, Ear, and Throat
    Hospital
Lenox Hill Hospital
Hofstra North Shore-LIJ School of Medicine
New York, New York

Richard K. Parrish II, MD (Question 20)
Associate Dean for Graduate Medical
    Education
Professor, Department of Ophthalmology
Bascom Palmer Eye Institute
University of Miami Miller School of
    Medicine
Designated Institutional Official
Jackson Memorial Hospital
Miami, Florida

Jody R. Piltz-Seymour, MD (Question 9)
Clinical Professor Ophthalmology
Perelman School of Medicine,
University of Pennsylvania
Director, Glaucoma Care Center, PC
Valley Eye Professionals
Huntingdon Valley, Pennsylvania

*Pradeep Ramulu, MD, PhD, MHS
    (Question 5)*
Associate Professor of Ophthalmology
Wilmer Eye Institute
Johns Hopkins University
Baltimore Maryland

Vineet Ratra, DNB, FRCS(Ed) (Question 46)
C-MER (Shenzhen) Dennis Lam Eye
    Hospital
Hong Kong, China

Robert Ritch, MD (Questions 24, 25)
Shelley and Steven Einhorn Distinguished
    Chair
Professor of Ophthalmology
Surgeon Director and Chief, Glaucoma
    Services
The New York Eye and Ear Infirmary
Founder, Medical Director and
Chairman, Scientific Advisory
    Board
The Glaucoma Foundation
New York, New York

Alan L. Robin, MD (Question 26)
Clinical Professor, Ophthalmology, University
    of Maryland
Adjunct Professor, Ophthalmology, University
    of Michigan
Associate Professor, Ophthalmology and
    International Health
Johns Hopkins University
Baltimore, Maryland

Hady Saheb, MD (Question 49)
McGill University Health Center
Department of Ophthalmology
Montreal, Canada

Leonard K. Seibold, MD (Question 48)
Department of Ophthalmology
University of Colorado School of Medicine
Aurora, Colorado

Bhavna P. Sheth, MD, MBA (Question 32)
Professor of Ophthalmology
Department of Ophthalmology
Medical College of Wisconsin Eye
    Institute
Milwaukee, Wisconsin

Paul A. Sidoti, MD (Question 43)
Professor of Ophthalmology
Deputy Chair for Clinical Affairs
Icahn School of Medicine at Mount Sinai
New York, New York

Kuldev Singh, MD, MPH (Question 2)
Professor of Ophthalmology
Director, Glaucoma Service
Stanford University School of Medicine
Stanford, California

Arthur J. Sit, MD, SM (Question 13)
Associate Professor
Department of Ophthalmology
College of Medicine
Mayo Clinic
Rochester, Minnesota

Alon Skaat, MD (Question 37)
Glaucoma Associates of New York
New York Eye and Ear Infirmary of Mount
    Sinai
New York, New York

Jeffrey R. SooHoo, MD (Question 48)
Department of Ophthalmology
University of Colorado School of
    Medicine
Aurora, Colorado

Angelo P. Tanna, MD (Question 8)
Vice Chairman, Department of
    Ophthalmology
Director, Glaucoma Service
Northwestern University
Feinberg School of Medicine
Chicago, Illinois

*Joshua C. Teichman, MD, MPH, FRCSC
    (Question 47)*
Cornea and External Disease
Cataract and Refractive Surgery
Oakville, Ontario, Canada

Celso Tello, MD (Question 24)
Professor and Chairman of Ophthalmology
Manhattan Eye, Ear, and Throat Hospital
Lenox Hill Hospital
Hofstra North Shore-LIJ School of
    Medicine
New York, New York

James C. Tsai, MD, MBA (Question 28)
The New York Eye and Ear Infirmary of
    Mount Sinai
Icahn School of Medicine at
    Mount Sinai
New York, New York

Reena S. Vaswani, MD (Question 11)
The New York Eye and Ear Infirmary of
    Mount Sinai
New York, New York

Martin Wand, MD (Question 36)
Clinical Professor of
    Ophthalmology
University of Connecticut School of
    Medicine
Consulting Ophthalmologists
Farmington, Connecticut

Sarah R. Wellik, MD (Question 31)
Associate Professor of
    Ophthalmology
Bascom Palmer Eye Institute
University of Miami Miller School of
    Medicine
Miami, Florida

Darrell WuDunn, MD, PhD (Question 27)
Professor and Residency Program
    Director
Eugene and Marilyn Glick Eye
    Institute
Department of Ophthalmology
Indiana University School of
    Medicine
Indianapolis, Indiana

Preface

Most clinicians routinely solicit advice from colleagues when confronted with a challenging patient. These "curbside consults" are an important part of the practice of medicine, and they serve to enhance the quality of care delivered. The advice is generally succinct, and it is based on knowledge, experience, and judgment. This book seeks to capture the essence of the "curbside consult."

The second edition of *Curbside Consultation in Glaucoma* has preserved the same format as the first edition. We have compiled 49 questions commonly encountered in clinical practice. The authors have provided answers that meet the four "Cs" of content—current (timely), concise (summarizing), credible (evidence based), and clinically relevant (practical). Half of the questions were retained from the first edition with updating by the authors. The other half consists of new questions introducing fresh content.

The book has been organized into 5 sections: General Principles, Glaucoma Diagnosis, General Management, Medical Therapy, and Laser and Incisional Glaucoma Surgery. Many aspects of the management of patients with glaucoma remain controversial. The authors have provided their viewpoints as experts in the field, but they should not be misinterpreted as a standard of care or absolute best approach.

We hope you enjoy this book and find it helpful in caring for your patients with glaucoma.

Steven J. Gedde, MD
Dale K. Heuer, MD
Richard A. Lewis, MD
Joseph F. Panarelli, MD

SECTION I

GENERAL PRINCIPLES

HOW FREQUENTLY DOES BLINDNESS DEVELOP AMONG PATIENTS WITH PRIMARY OPEN-ANGLE GLAUCOMA? WITH OCULAR HYPERTENSION?

Philip P. Chen, MD

Definition and Scope

The United States Social Security Administration defines *legal blindness* as, in the better eye, visual acuity of 20/200 or worse or visual field (VF) constriction to 20 degrees or less with the Humphrey size III stimulus at 10 dB or the Goldmann size III4e stimulus. Unless otherwise specified, this definition will be used for all further references to *blindness* in this chapter. Population-based, cross-sectional studies that examined thousands of individuals in developed countries (United States, Ireland, the Netherlands, and Australia) comprised mostly of Whites have reported the prevalence of bilateral blindness from open-angle glaucoma (OAG) to be approximately 3% to 7%.[1]

Clinical Studies in Patients With Open-Angle Glaucoma

UNTREATED PATIENTS

An untreated African-derived population on the Caribbean island of St. Lucia with definite or suspected OAG was examined 10 years later and found to have progression to end-stage VF loss (defined as an Advanced Glaucoma Intervention Study [AGIS] score of 18 to 20 on a 0 to 20 scale) in one eye of 16% and in both eyes of 9%.[2] Notably, almost 60% of eyes with end-stage glaucoma after 10 years had no or minimal VF loss at initial testing, indicating fairly rapid progression, up to 2 to 3 dB/y. Progression was associated with age but not intraocular pressure (IOP).

Gedde SJ, ed. *Curbside Consultation in Glaucoma:*
49 Clinical Questions, Second Edition (pp 3–6)
© 2015 Taylor & Francis Group

Treated Patients

Studies investigating blindness in patients with OAG are summarized in Table 1-1.[2–7] Among older studies, Grant and Burke[1] noted a preponderance of Black patients among those blind from glaucoma. Hattenhauer et al[3] performed a retrospective study of 295 patients in Olmsted County, Minnesota, who had been diagnosed between 1965 and 1980. Most patients had been followed using kinetic perimetry. Among 100 White patients diagnosed with classic glaucoma (based on at least 2 of the following at the time of diagnosis: elevated IOP, optic disc damage, and VF loss), the respective estimates for unilateral and bilateral blindness at 20 years were 54% and 22%.

More recent studies that followed patients tested with automated perimetry and benefiting from advances in glaucoma diagnosis, medications, and surgical treatments have shown variable rates of blindness. Chen[4] studied 186 patients (82% White) with treated OAG diagnosed in 1975 or later. These patients were diagnosed relatively early (mean age at diagnosis of 60 years) and treated primarily by glaucoma subspecialists. The Kaplan-Meier estimate at 15 years was 14.6% for unilateral blindness and 6.4% for bilateral blindness. The estimate at 15 years for bilateral visual acuity of 20/200 or worse from glaucoma was 4.1%.

Several European studies have examined the true lifetime risk of blindness among patients with glaucoma identified by death certificate. These studies report variable results with unilateral and bilateral blindness rates of 6.6% to 38% and 0% to 14%, respectively, at up to 20 years by Kaplan-Meier analysis (see Table 1-1).[5–7] Notably, Peters et al[7] found blindness rates of 38% in one eye and 13.5% bilaterally at 20 years, although the studied cohort was older at diagnosis (74 years), had more advanced disease at diagnosis (presenting worse-eye VF mean deviation of –11.8 dB), and had higher rates of pseudoexfoliation glaucoma (40%) than did patients in Chen's study.[4]

Advances in filtering surgery have also benefited patients. The AGIS reported on 776 eyes (581 patients) randomized to 1 of 2 surgical treatment sequences and found the cumulative incidence of blindness (defined as an AGIS VF score of 18–20) at 10 years to be 15.0% in Black patients and 8.6% in White patients.[8] Landers et al[9] reported similar findings in a long-term review of trabeculectomy, with 15% of eyes blind at 20 years. These rates are lower than data reported from the Olmsted County study (46% at 10 years), although those patients had surgery between 1965 and 1994.

Risk factors for blindness identified in these studies have included older age, worse VF loss at diagnosis, noncompliance, pseudoexfoliation, and difficulty with IOP control.[1,4,6,7,9]

Ocular Hypertension

Few studies have specifically considered the long-term outcomes of patients diagnosed initially with ocular hypertension (OHT) using modern diagnostic tests. Recently, Gestel et al[10] used a Markov model with data from a systematic literature review to estimate that the 15-year risk of unilateral blindness was less than 10%.

What Is the Goal of Treatment?

The goal of glaucoma treatment is the preservation of vision and vision-related quality of life throughout the patient's lifetime. I reassure patients diagnosed with OHT or early OAG that worsening to blindness is uncommon if adherence with treatment and follow-up is good. Younger patients obviously must be informed that predicting disease course over many decades is difficult. The prognosis is more guarded in patients with pseudoexfoliation, moderately advanced glaucoma,

Table 1-1

Summary of Studies on Blindness From Open-Angle Glaucoma*

	Wilson†	Grant and Burke	Hattenhauer	Chen	Ang	Forsmann	Peters
Year published	2002	1982	1998	2003	2007	2007	2013
Setting	Population-based	Clinic	Clinic	Clinic	Clinic/death records	Clinic/death records	Clinic/death records
Type	OHT + OAG	OHT + POAG	OHT + POAG/POAG	OAG	OAG	OHT/OAG	OAG
N	155	131	295/100	186	121	106	592
Year of diagnosis	1990	≤1960	1965 to 1980	≥1975	≥1970	≥1976	≥1977
% PXG	0	N/A	8.5	14	0	37	40
Blind 1 eye	16% at 10 years	37% at 20 years	27% at 20 years/54% at 20 years‡	14% at 15 years	6.6% at 7 years[1]	15% at 15 years[2]	38% at 20 yrs[3]
Mean follow-up (years)	10	20+	15	9	7	10	11

*OHT indicates ocular hypertension; POAG, primary open-angle glaucoma; OAG, open-angle glaucoma; PXG, pseudoexfoliation glaucoma.
† Untreated, African-derived.
‡ 27% for OHT + POAG, 54% for POAG only.
[1] 20/200 or worse, or 'severe visual field defect' and 20/50 or worse
[2] 20/200 or worse, or VF < 10 degrees
[3] 20/400 or worse, or VF < 10 degrees

or in whom IOP control is difficult, as well as in those who are nonadherent. Greater vigilance and more aggressive treatment may be necessary for long-term preservation of vision in these patients.

References

1. Chen PP. Risk and risk factors for blindness from glaucoma. *Curr Opin Ophthalmol.* 2004;15:107-111.
2. Wilson MR, Kosoko O, Cowan CL Jr, et al. Progression of visual field loss in untreated glaucoma patients and glaucoma suspects in St. Lucia, West Indies. *Am J Ophthalmol.* 2002;134:399-405.
3. Hattenhauer MG, Johnson DH, Ing HH, et al. The probability of blindness from open-angle glaucoma. *Ophthalmology.* 1998;105:2099-2104.
4. Chen PP. Blindness among patients with treated open angle glaucoma. *Ophthalmology.* 2003;110:726-733.
5. Ang GS, Eke T. Lifetime visual prognosis for patients with primary open-angle glaucoma. *Eye.* 2007;21:604-608.
6. Forsman E, Kivela T, Vesti E. Lifetime visual disability in open-angle glaucoma and ocular hypertension. *J Glaucoma.* 2007;16:313-319.
7. Peters D, Bengtsson B, Heijl A. Lifetime risk of blindness in open-angle glaucoma. *Am J Ophthalmol.* 2013;156:724-730.
8. The AGIS Investigators. Advanced Glaucoma Intervention Study (AGIS): 13. Comparison of treatment outcomes within race: 10-year results. *Ophthalmology.* 2004;111:651-664.
9. Landers J, Martin K, Sharkies N, et al. A twenty-year follow-up study of trabeculectomy: risk factors and outcomes. *Ophthalmology.* 2012;119:694-702.
10. Gestel AV, Webers CA, Beckers HJ, et al. Ocular hypertension and the risk of blindness [published online March 20, 2013]. *J Glaucoma.*

DOES REDUCING INTRAOCULAR PRESSURE REALLY PREVENT THE DEVELOPMENT AND PROGRESSION OF GLAUCOMA?

Kuldev Singh, MD, MPH

The only modifiable risk factor in glaucoma care is intraocular pressure (IOP), and thus the only way a practitioner can reduce the risk of glaucoma development and progression is by lowering IOP. The goal of glaucoma therapy is to slow the rate of disease progression to a rate consistent with functionally useful vision for the remainder of a patient's life. Given the redundancy in the visual system, every retinal ganglion cell does not have to be preserved for a patient to be able to read or drive. It is well known that the lower the IOP among individuals in a given population, the lower the likelihood of being diagnosed with glaucoma at a particular time.[1,2] It has also been shown that lowering IOP reduces the likelihood of developing glaucoma and slows the rate of glaucoma progression.[3,4]

Disease Development

The Ocular Hypertension Treatment Study (OHTS) showed that even if the desired 20% IOP lowering was achieved, approximately 5% of study participants receiving medical therapy to achieve such reduction developed glaucoma over 5 years.[3] Could this rate have been reduced to zero had IOP been lowered further? Probably not, and there is no good evidence to support a hypothesis that the risk of developing open-angle glaucoma can be completely eliminated by lowering IOP. Given the existence of nonmodifiable risk factors for glaucoma development and the influence of aging on retinal ganglion cell health, it is unlikely that even reducing IOP to very low levels can always prevent the development of glaucoma in all patients.

Gedde SJ, ed. *Curbside Consultation in Glaucoma:*
49 Clinical Questions, Second Edition (pp 7–9)
© 2015 Taylor & Francis Group

Disease Progression

In some and perhaps most patients, progression of glaucoma, like most chronic diseases, can only be slowed rather than completely stabilized. A patient may have a visual field test that is statistically unchanged from prior such tests. Similarly, examination of the optic nerve may reveal no discernible change from prior photographs or imaging scans. In such situations, we can say that the visual field or optic nerve appears stable, but we cannot state with certainty that the disease is stable rather than progressing at a very slow rate that is not detectable by the clinician. The tools that we use to determine glaucoma progression do not have the resolution necessary to determine all meaningful change. As with the development of glaucoma, there are risk factors for progression not related to IOP. It would be naïve to assume that lowering IOP, one of several risk factors for glaucoma progression, can completely halt the death of retinal ganglion cells over time in patients with glaucoma.

Target Intraocular Pressure

The IOP–primary open-angle glaucoma (POAG) relationship is not understood well enough to strongly support the target IOP concept[5]; nonetheless, a target IOP may be conceptually useful to many practitioners when initiating glaucoma therapy. It has the potential, however, to mislead patients and practitioners into thinking that if the IOP is above an arbitrary target goal, glaucoma will progress, and if it is below that goal, the disease process will stabilize. Savvy practitioners do not overstate the utility of this concept and recognize that setting a target IOP must be a dynamic process in which the target IOP may need adjustment based on multiple factors, including disease status, patient age and life expectancy, treatment efficacy and adverse effects, and likelihood of surgical success and complications.

All things being equal, the lower the IOP, the slower the rate of glaucoma progression. However, there is no good evidence to suggest that there is a particular IOP level at which glaucoma progression completely stops and the determination of the IOP-POAG relationship cannot be prospectively determined for the individual patient at this time.

A post hoc associative analysis of pooled data from the Advanced Glaucoma Intervention Study (AGIS) suggested that if IOP could be kept below 18 mm Hg at all 6-month study visits, glaucoma might be stabilized; the mean IOP of the AGIS participants whose IOP met that criterion was approximately 12 mm Hg.[6] It is noteworthy that 12 mm Hg represents the mean of all individual patient means in this subgroup, and some with all IOPs under 18 mm Hg had mean IOPs higher than 12 mm Hg. Another limitation of this analysis was that some patients in this subgroup had improvement of visual fields, whereas others showed worsening, such that the average showed no change over 8 years. It is well known that visual field tests show substantial fluctuation, with the OHTS revealing that approximately 85% of patients thought to have progression on a single visual field showed no significant change on subsequent testing.[7] Overall, the AGIS results do not confirm that an IOP above or below 12 mm Hg guarantees disease progression or stability, respectively.

What We Might Tell Our Patients

Lowering IOP decreases the likelihood of our ocular hypertensive patients developing glaucoma and our glaucoma patients showing progression based on our present examination techniques. Lowering IOP does not, however, ensure that glaucoma progression will stop. Fortunately, slowing progression of the disease by lowering IOP, particularly if the disease is diagnosed sufficiently early, will commonly allow our patients to maintain functional vision over their entire lifetimes. In the future, other therapies for glaucoma besides IOP lowering may be available to further slow glaucoma progression, but a treatment that will generally halt glaucoma progression will likely not be available any time soon.

References

1. Sommer A, Tielsch JM, Katz J, et al. Relationship between intraocular pressure and primary open angle glaucoma among White and Black Americans: the Baltimore Eye Survey. *Arch Ophthalmol.* 1991;109:1090-1095.
2. Tielsch JM, Katz J, Singh K, et al. A population-based evaluation of glaucoma screening: the Baltimore Eye Survey. *Am J Epidemiol.* 1991;134:1102-1110.
3. Kass MA, Heuer DK, Higginbotham EJ, et al. The Ocular Hypertension Treatment Study. *Arch Ophthalmol.* 2002;120:701-713.
4. Leske MC, Heijl A, Hussein M, et al, for the Early Manifest Glaucoma Trial Group. Factors for glaucoma progression and the effect of treatment: the Early Manifest Glaucoma Trial. *Arch Ophthalmol.* 2003;121:48-56.
5. Singh K, Spaeth G, Zimmerman T, Minckler D. Target IOP: glaucoma's holy grail. *Ophthalmology.* 2000;107:629-630.
6. AGIS Investigators. The relationship between control of intraocular pressure and visual field deterioration. *Am J Ophthalmol.*2000;130:429-440.
7. Keltner JL, Johnson CA, Quigg JM, et al. Confirmation of visual field abnormalities in the Ocular Hypertension Treatment Study. *Arch Ophthalmol.* 2000;118:1187-1194.

Are Vascular Factors Involved in the Pathogenesis of Glaucoma?

Douglas R. Anderson, MD, FARVO

Historical Perspective

As optic disc changes are clinically the most prominent fundus feature in glaucoma, it has been assumed that the pathogenic process must be located there. Early support for this hypothesis was that the optic disc, unlike the retina and the rest of the optic nerve, derives its arterial supply from branches of the posterior ciliary arteries that pass through the choroid to enter the optic nerve head. Unlike the retina, the choroidal blood flow is affected by the intraocular pressure (IOP), a physiologic feature assumed to include the optic disc.[1] The choroidal arterial filling during angiography occurs in patches corresponding to the regions supplied by each of the numerous choroidal arteriolar branches of the posterior ciliary artery. The region in each patch furthest from the feeding arteriole might be a "watershed" zone more vulnerable to any challenge to blood flow.[1] Often, the boundary between two patches bisects the optic disc vertically, and it was hypothesized that this explained the particular susceptibility of the upper and lower poles of the optic disc, resulting in damage to the part of the disc serving the upper and lower arcuate regions and the peripheral temporal retina, corresponding to the typical location of field defects in glaucoma.

An alternate plausible hypothesis was that the damage occurred in the retina. In particular, the elongated radial peripapillary capillaries that occupy the retinal nerve fiber layer might be more susceptible to compression by elevated IOP and produce ischemia due to their longer course from arteriole to venule.[2] Moreover, they are most numerous in the upper and lower arcuate regions, corresponding to the typical location of the nerve fiber bundle and nasal visual field defects.

Finally, some felt it likely that direct mechanical damage to the physical structure of the disc was responsible for the development of deep cupping and that anatomical features of the lamina cribrosa accounted for the typical location of damage to axons passing through that region. It was noted that the openings in the lamina cribrosa were larger near the poles of the disc, while those

Gedde SJ, ed. *Curbside Consultation in Glaucoma:*
49 Clinical Questions, Second Edition (pp 11–14)
© 2015 Taylor & Francis Group

on the temporal side were smaller, accommodating the passage of the smaller axons from the macula, and perhaps more resistant to mechanical influence.

Although speculative, each hypothesis had both a physiologic rationale as well as an explanation of the characteristic location of nerve damage and visual field loss in chronic glaucoma. Suggestive evidence for each was collected in the years following introduction of the hypotheses.

Laboratory Studies

Demonstration in monkeys that rapid axonal transport (to be distinguished from slow axonal flow, which results in disc swelling [papilledema][3-5]) is impaired by elevated IOP was the first physiologic abnormality to be demonstrated that resulted from IOP.[6] It was later shown that blockage was the result of impaired blood flow rather than a mechanical effect of the lamina cribrosa,[7] although this explanation was not universally accepted. Interruption of retrograde axonal transport, if prolonged enough, is expected to produce ganglion cell apoptosis because nerve growth factor, responsible for maintaining viability of the ganglion cell, comes from the lateral geniculate body by this retrograde transport. Rather quickly, apoptosis of ganglion cells in experimental glaucoma was shown, along with quite a cascade of changes in the molecular physiology, affecting axons, neurons, and support tissues, such as the astroglia.[8]

Moreover, the lamina cribrosa becomes bowed backward more than normal, and its insertion into the sclera is displaced backward to insert into the pia mater, presumably with remodeling of the connective tissue elements.[9,10] The exit canal through the sclera may widen, at least posteriorly, and these changes in the lamina cribrosa and sclera account for the glaucomatous excavation of the disc, whereas simple loss of axons, as occurs in other types of optic atrophy, does not typically have acquired cupping. Opinions differ as to whether the thinning and deterioration of the lamina cribrosa results from the same ischemia that affects the neural tissue of the optic nerve head (perhaps with reperfusion injury[8,11] if ischemia is intermittent) or whether the mechanical changes in the lamina cribrosa affect the configuration of the capillary bed to help produce ischemia.

What is clear is that whatever initiates the damage, there is a cascade of numerous consequences in the microphysiology and cellular biology in the affected tissues.[8]

Clinical Evidence

The IOP raises the venous pressure at the exit point from the eye, reducing the arteriovenous pressure difference that pushes blood through the vascular channels. The flow is controlled by a complex mechanism called *autoregulation*, meaning the flow is regulated according to local conditions such as metabolic need when the tissue is active or there are changes in either the venous pressure or arterial pressure. This control is accomplished by complex regulation of the diameters of the arteries, capillaries, and veins in order to control not only the volume of blood flow but also the intraluminal pressure of the capillaries (to prevent edema).[12]

Not only the IOP but also the capacity for regulation may vary from moment to moment. For example, if there is hypovolemia due to excessive blood loss, all vascular beds of the body may dilate in an effort to maintain blood flow, and the reserve capacity for further dilation in face of another challenge (such as IOP) may be compromised. The clinical import of this concept is that just as IOP, when measured at an office visit, may not represent all other times between visits, any measure of blood flow in the office may not represent what happens during sleep or during exercise at high altitudes when skiing. Thus, it is the determination of the reserve capacity for regulation that will be of clinical importance, when a method for doing so is developed.

What is known from clinical studies is that a certain percentage of people do not seem to have much capacity to regulate at all (2 of 10 in one study[13]), and this may explain why some eyes withstand ocular hypertension, while others with an abnormal IOP develop glaucoma. Other forms of vascular dysregulation are manifest in certain patients with glaucoma, particularly those with slight elevation of IOP or an IOP distinctly within the statistically normal range of healthy eyes. Such dysregulation (or vasospastic disease) can be found by testing the response of fingernail capillary beds to cold[14] or by the patient reporting a history of a tendency for cold hands and feet (wearing socks at night while sleeping), auras with migraine, lack of thirst, low blood pressure, and so on. Another mechanism for limited regulatory reserve is occlusive arterial disease (atherosclerosis), and stenosis may cause the more distal vessels to dilate markedly, leaving little reserve for dilation to overcome another challenge, such as IOP, and thus little therapeutic benefit to lowering the IOP.[15] It is important to note that even normal IOP raises venous pressure above orbital venous pressure and is hence a challenge to circulation, accounting for some cases of normal-tension glaucoma, and that reducing the challenge (lowering IOP) is helpful in most cases.

On the basis of evidence that blood flow is at least part of the problem, clinicians may pay attention to "ocular perfusion pressure," the difference between arterial pressure estimated from the brachial artery and venous pressure in the eye designated as having IOP.[16] Low blood pressure occurs in those with vascular dysregulation during all times of day, during sleep, and at the time of cardiovascular crisis (shock),[17] which may produce a nonprogressive form of normal-tension glaucoma. However, the relationship between "ocular perfusion pressure" and glaucomatous pathogenesis is impure due to dynamic physiologic changes in the cardiovascular system that may preserve blood flow to vital organs during challenging times.[8,16]

Thus, the clinical evidence to support vascular contributions to the etiology of glaucoma includes the finding of patients with a history of severe (but nonlethal) shock, a frequent finding of vascular dysregulation (particularly among those with glaucoma at lower IOPs), and perhaps patients with atherosclerotic disease (who may not be helped much by lowering of IOP).[15] It seems that the optic nerve head has a somewhat unique vascular physiology, which makes it susceptible to outside influence such as vasospasm and glaucomatous disease results depending on the regulatory reserve in face of these other conditions and the additional challenge posed by IOP. At present, we can lower the IOP but have not yet discovered how to affect the fundamental anatomic and physiologic factors, vascular and nonvascular, that make some eyes develop glaucoma (while others have abnormally high IOP without having damage). Whether there are fundamental structural abnormalities of the lamina cribrosa that also make or contribute to the nerve's susceptibility is unknown but is under study.

References

1. Hayreh SS. The blood supply of the optic nerve head and the evaluation of it—myth and reality. *Prog Retin Eye Res.* 2001;20(5):563-593.
2. Alterman M, Henkind P. Radial peripapillary capillaries of the retina, II: possible role in Bjerrum scotoma. *Br J Ophthalmol.* 1968;52:26-31.
3. Radius RL, Anderson DR. Morphology of axonal transport abnormalities in primate eyes. *Br J Ophthalmol.* 1981;65:767-777.
4. Anderson DR. Axonal transport in the retina and optic nerve. In: Glaser JS, ed. *Neuro-Ophthalmology Symposium of the University of Miami and the Bascom Palmer Eye Institute.* Vol 9. St Louis, MO: CV Mosby; 1977:140-153.
5. Anderson DR. Papilledema and axonal transport. In: Thompson H, Daroff R, Frisen L, Glaser JS, Sanders MD, eds. *Topics in Neuro-Ophthalmology.* Baltimore, MD: Williams & Wilkins; 1979:184-189.
6. Anderson DR, Hendrickson A. Effect of intraocular pressure on rapid axoplasmic transport in monkey optic nerve. *Invest Ophthalmol Vis Sci.* 1974;13:771-783.
7. Sossi N, Anderson DR. Blockage of axonal transport in optic nerve induced by elevation of intraocular pressure: effect of arterial hypertension induced by angiotensin I. *Arch Ophthalmol.* 1983;101:94-97.

8. Mozaffarieh M, Flammer J. What is the present pathogenetic concept of glaucomatous optic neuropathy? *Surv Ophthalmol.* 2007;52:S162-S173.

9. Burgoyne CF, Downs JC, Bellezza AJ, Suh JK, Hart RT. The optic nerve head as a biomechanical structure: a new paradigm for understanding the role of IOP-related stress and strain in the pathophysiology of glaucomatous optic nerve head damage. *Prog Retin Eye Res.* 2005;24(1):39-73.

10. Roberts MD, Grau V, Grimm J, et al. Remodeling of the connective tissue microarchitecture of the lamina cribrosa in early experimental glaucoma. *Invest Ophthalmol Vis Sci.* 2009;50:681-690.

11. Flammer J. Glaucomatous optic neuropathy: a reperfusion injury [in German]. *Klin Monatsbl Augenheilkd.* 2001;218:290-291.

12. Anderson DR. Glaucoma, capillaries, and pericytes, 1: blood flow regulation. *Ophthalmologica.* 1996;210:257-262.

13. Pillunat LE, Anderson DR, Knighton RW, Joos KM, Feuer WJ. Autoregulation in human optic nerve head circulation in response to increased intraocular pressure. *Exp Eye Res.* 1997;64:737-744.

14. Drance SM, Douglas GR, Wijsman K, Schulzer M, Britton RJ. Response of blood flow to warm and cold in normal and low-tension glaucoma patients. *Am J Ophthalmol.* 1988;105(1):35-39.

15. Anderson DR, Drance SM, Schulzer M. Factors that predict the benefit of lowering intraocular pressure in normal tension glaucoma. *Am J Ophthalmol.* 2003;136:820-829.

16. Costa VP, Harris A, Anderson DR, et al. Ocular perfusion pressure in glaucoma. *Acta Ophthalmol.* 2014;92(4):e252-e266.

17. Drance SM. Shock-induced optic neuropathy: a cause of non-progressive glaucoma. *N Engl J Med.* 1973;288:392.

What Are the Most Frequent Causes of Glaucoma-Related Medical Malpractice Suits? What Can I Do to Minimize My Risk?

E. Randy Craven, MD, FACS

You might worry about a patient with glaucoma wanting to sue you because your recall system did not send out the letter last month for the glaucoma follow-up. However, I have found that it is usually not the missed appointments that cause suits; it is more frequently miscommunication that leads to the patient suing. Most malpractice suits for glaucoma are related to our surgical care of glaucoma, our care causing glaucoma (such as from using steroids for blepharitis or from retained lens material after cataract surgery),[2] or our failure to recognize glaucoma progression (Figure 4-1). Patients who want to sue us do so because of a perceived lack of caring and/or collaboration in the delivery of their care. Issues that have been identified with malpractice suits include perceived unavailability, discounting patient and/or family concerns, poor delivery of information, and lack of understanding the patient's and/or family's perspective.[1,3] In busy ophthalmology practices, you need to have a safety valve should problems arise. How you handle the patient after a problem is even more crucial. Carefully designed office "SWAT" teams can help manage potential litigious patients. Referrals can help you avoid litigation.

When you ask plaintiffs why they are suing the defendant doctor, a feeling of something hidden or not revealed almost always emerges. For instance, if you did a trabeculectomy and the patient had a low intraocular pressure (IOP) right after the surgery and you did not mention that he or she should be cautious with bending or stooping and then has a hemorrhage, it is difficult to repair that missed communication. This is why I try to have standard scripts that I tell patients who have glaucoma. You should attempt to achieve consistency in what you tell patients so your staff also picks up on this. For instance, if someone is to return in a few months for a visual field, I look at the request for testing as an opportunity to educate the patient. "Mrs. Jones, you are coming back in 3 months to see me because we are monitoring your glaucoma. What we are looking for is stability of your glaucoma damage. As you know, some of your peripheral vision has been lost, so we are going to recheck your visual field. I hope you understand how important it is for me to help you

Gedde SJ, ed. *Curbside Consultation in Glaucoma:*
49 Clinical Questions, Second Edition (pp 15-17)
© 2015 Taylor & Francis Group

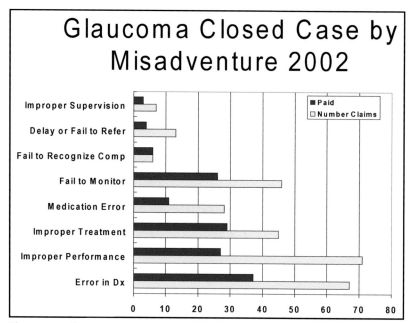

Figure 4-1. Glaucoma closed case by misadventure, 2002.

keep your vision." If a patient is undergoing glaucoma filtration surgery, I will check the IOP on the first day and reinforce what concerns I have. For instance, if the IOP is low, I will say, "Mrs. Jones, the pressure reduction from the surgery has been successful for now. Time will tell how successful. This is why I need to see you. Now what I need you to do is to use the drops and be cautious with bending or lifting. When the pressure is low, you might have a hemorrhage. Once the pressure goes up there is less of a risk."

Recruit the patient's family and your staff to help keep the patient informed and from feeling frustrated. I like to ask patients for whom I am scheduling surgery if they would like anyone to come with them when we discuss their surgery. "You know, two heads are better than one." Even more essential is that your records system supports these discussions. Without a written record, we will have difficulty getting any jury to believe we did what we said we did. Teach your staff that you are really talking to them a lot of the time, and they need to pick up on your phrases that key them to record what you are saying. For instance, if you say, "Mrs. Jones, what I plan to do is . . . ," this tells the scribe where it goes on the record. Even more important, if you have a problem or something that could lead to a problem, you should ask the family or friends to come in to hear the discussion and to help ask questions the patient may have forgotten to ask or was afraid to ask.

Glaucoma suits account for less than 10% of ophthalmologic malpractice claims, but the settlements can exceed $1 million. The data used to review glaucoma claims come from either the Physician Insurers Association of America (PIAA) or from the data held by the Ophthalmic Mutual Insurance Company (OMIC). As of the end of 2004, there had been 6069 ophthalmic malpractice claims reported over 20 years. Of these, about 6% (350 claims) were related to glaucoma. OMIC had about 150 cases with glaucoma as the (or a) leading diagnosis in the case by the end of 2002. Some cases might have 2 diagnoses, such as cataract (with surgery) and secondary glaucoma. Because of the length of time required for vision loss to occur in most patients, you would think that the lawsuits related to glaucoma are usually from patients who have seen the doctor for years and the diagnosis or progression was missed. With all the new nerve-imaging devices and visual field technology, the patients should expect us to pick up and monitor the glaucoma. A large subset of patients who sue are those who experience a sudden loss of vision or eye function after surgery. Taking your time when consenting a patient and being truthful about your postoperative concerns as discussed previously can help minimize patient dissatisfaction and potentially avoid future suits.

References

1. Ambady N, Laplante D, Nguyen T, et al. Surgeons' tone of voice: a clue to malpractice history. *Surgery.* 2002;132:5-9.
2. Craven, ER. Risk management issues in glaucoma. *Surv Ophthalmol.* 1996;40:459-462.
3. Vincent C, Young M, Phillips A. Why do people sue doctors? A study of patients and relatives taking legal action. *Lancet.* 1994;343:1609-1613.

HOW DOES GLAUCOMA AFFECT QUALITY OF LIFE? WHY DOES IT MATTER?

Pradeep Ramulu, MD, PhD, MHS

Preserving quality of life is the goal of glaucoma management, and many studies describe how glaucoma affects the patient. But how do we use this research in clinical practice? In this section, we describe how the impact of glaucoma varies with disease severity and illustrate how to use this information in specific clinical scenarios.

Scenario 1: What Is the Impact of Refusing IOP-Lowering Surgery?

It is frequently difficult to convince patients that they require a surgery with no possibility of improving their vision and some possibility of worsening it. In such discussions, it is critical to tell patients what will happen if surgery is not pursued. Early in my career, I told patients that without surgery, there was the risk of going totally blind, or I vaguely described how their vision "would get worse." Patients with minimal vision loss, with good reason, found it hard to believe that they would go blind without surgery, while vague descriptions of "worse vision" made it hard for others to accept the risks of surgery.

Many studies describe how behavior, function, and quality of life differ across a range of visual field (VF) loss, and these studies can be used to describe to patients the impact of greater visual field loss (Table 5-1 summarizes the impact of a 5-dB difference in the mean deviation [MD] of the better eye). This information can then be combined with information regarding how quickly VF damage is occurring. The VF MD in untreated primary open-angle glaucoma (POAG) worsens, on average, at 1 dB/y (although patients with severe intraocular pressure [IOP] elevation, pseudoexfoliation, or documented rapid progression are likely to progress much faster).

Gedde SJ, ed. *Curbside Consultation in Glaucoma:*
49 Clinical Questions, Second Edition (pp 19–21)
© 2015 Taylor & Francis Group

Table 5-1
Quantifiable Deficits Associated with Greater Visual Field Loss in Glaucoma

Functional/Quality of Life Metric	Deficit Associated With a 5-dB Decrement in the Mean Deviation of the Better-Seeing Eye
Speed of book reading	11% slower
Daily steps	10% fewer
Time spent in moderate/vigorous physical activity	22% less
Odds of not leaving home on a given day	24% higher
Fear of falling	0.47 logits worse
Driving cessation	2-fold higher odds
Greater driving restriction	1.6-fold higher odds
Injuring oneself from a fall	35% more likely

Thus, if my patient's VF MD is progressing at 1 dB/y in the better eye, I would tell her that in 5 years, she would read 10% slower,[1] walk 10% less,[2] engage in 20% less physical activity,[2] have a 2-fold higher odds of no longer driving (assuming she is still driving now),[3] be 25% more likely to not leave the home on a given day, and be 35% more likely to injure herself from a fall.[4] The risks of surgery and likelihood of avoiding these sequelae can then be discussed in this context.

Scenario 2: Should I (or My Loved One) Stop Driving?

Driving licensure guidelines are often vague and subject to considerable interpretation, and therefore I have avoided making recommendations solely based on whether a patient meets the visual requirements for driving. For example, many states specify the degrees of VF required to drive without specifying the target used in testing. Even when a specific test object/pattern is specified, there are no guidelines for translating field results into degrees of VF. These issues are compounded by a general lack of doctor/technician expertise with evaluating the VF outside the central 30 degrees (ie, using Esterman or Goldmann VFs).

Research has suggested that crash risks increase with severity of VF loss, although other studies found no clear association between glaucoma and crash rates. These disparate results likely reflect the fact that many glaucoma patients stop or significantly restrict their driving. My clinical approach has been to use published driving cessation patterns as a guide to whether or not patients should consider stopping driving. At a level of damage where one-third of patients with glaucoma have stopped driving (MD = –10 dB), I broach the topic of driving cessation and encourage a transition toward a lifestyle where driving is not required. At a level of VF loss where most patients are no longer driving (MD worse than –15 dB in the better-seeing eye), I recommend that patients stop driving and will generally not sign paperwork authorizing them to drive unless they pass a road test with a certified road instructor (a service not covered by insurance, unfortunately).

Scenario 3: How Can I Help My Patients With Advanced Disease?

You will, of course, monitor their VFs and control their IOP to preserve vision. But these patients are reading slower, falling more, and living in social isolation, and further IOP lowering will not help any of this. As ophthalmologists, we are generally not trained how to optimize reading, mobility, and function in those with low vision, but it is our responsibility to get our patients to specialists who can. We need to manage their disease to ensure that their future vision is no worse than today, and we must get our patients to low-vision specialists, occupational therapists, and orientation and mobility specialists to optimize how they function now. Indeed, studies show that intensive low-vision therapy can greatly reduce difficulty with multiple types of tasks. Thus, in patients with advanced, stable disease, visits to the glaucoma specialist should be well balanced with visits to visual rehabilitation specialists.

References

1. Ramulu PY, Swenor BK, Jefferys JL, Friedman DS, Rubin GS. Difficulty with out-loud and silent reading in glaucoma. *Invest Ophthalmol Vis Sci.* 2013;54(1):666-672.
2. Ramulu PY, Maul E, Hochberg C, Chan ES, Ferrucci L, Friedman DS. Real-world assessment of walking and physical activity in glaucoma using an accelerometer. *Ophthalmology.* 2012;119(6):1159-1166.
3. Ramulu PY, West SK, Munoz B, Jampel HD, Friedman DS. Driving cessation and driving limitation in glaucoma: the Salisbury Eye Evaluation project. *Ophthalmology.* 2009;116(10):1846-1853.
4. Black AA, Wood JM, Lovie-Kitchin JE. Inferior field loss increases rate of falls in older adults with glaucoma. *Optom Vis Sci.* 2011;88(11):1275-1282.

SECTION II

GLAUCOMA DIAGNOSIS

HOW SHOULD I CLINICALLY EXAMINE THE OPTIC NERVE?

Felipe A. Medeiros, MD, PhD

The most important characteristic of the glaucomatous process is the change that occurs in the optic nerve. As the axons of the retinal ganglion cells are lost, changes occur in the appearance of the retinal nerve fiber layer (RNFL) and optic disc that often precede the development of visual field defects. Therefore, it is important for the clinician to be familiar with the characteristic signs of glaucoma in the optic nerve. Even in the presence of visual field defects, progression of optic disc damage may occur without any detectable evidence of functional deterioration.

With regard to the technique of optic nerve examination, I usually perform an initial evaluation with the slit lamp using a 78-D Volk lens. A 60-D lens is also useful, although 90-D lenses may not provide sufficient magnification to fully appreciate all the details of the optic nerve. Direct ophthalmoscopy techniques do not provide the necessary stereopsis to adequately evaluate the extension of areas of rim thinning and cupping. After this initial evaluation, I usually obtain stereophotographs of the optic nerve so that I have an objective documentation to compare to at future follow-up visits. It is important to realize that a description of the optic nerve examination using only a simple measure such as the cup/disc ratio is insufficient for this purpose. Even a good optic nerve drawing is of limited value when comparing examinations over time. Glaucomatous changes in the optic nerve generally occur slowly over several years, and even well-drawn representations or detailed descriptions of the optic nerve can be insufficient to detect small increments of glaucomatous progression. In addition, assessment of the structural characteristics of the optic nerve, such as the cup/disc ratio, is subjective and can vary widely among different examiners. Objective recording of the appearance of the optic disc is therefore essential.

Evaluation of the optic nerve in patients who have or are suspected of having glaucoma should follow a systematic approach.[1] The examiner should have a sequence of steps to follow so that no important sign will be missed. We have described a set of 5 steps to facilitate evaluation of the optic nerve in clinical practice, which are known as the "5 Rs":

Gedde SJ, ed. *Curbside Consultation in Glaucoma:*
49 Clinical Questions, Second Edition (pp 25–30)
© 2015 Taylor & Francis Group

Figure 6-1. The first step in examining the optic nerve is identifying the scleral ring and the limits and size of the optic disc.

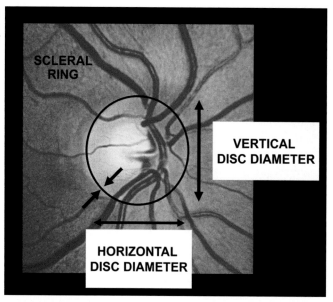

Figure 6-2. The size of the optic disc cup varies with the size of the optic disc. In healthy individuals, large discs tend to have large cups and small discs tend to have small cups.

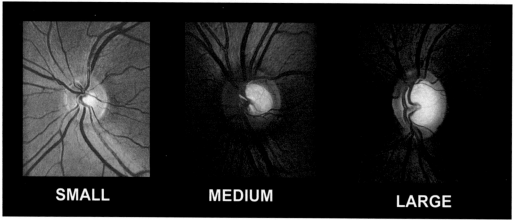

1. Observe the scleral **R**ing to identify the limits of the optic disc and to evaluate its size.
2. Identify the size of the **R**im.
3. Examine the **R**etinal nerve fiber layer.
4. Examine the **R**egion outside the optic disc for parapapillary atrophy.
5. Look for **R**etinal and optic disc hemorrhages.

In step 1, the evaluation of the optic disc starts with identification of the scleral ring and the limits of the optic disc (Figure 6-1). This allows the examiner to assess the size of the optic disc and how it relates to the neuroretinal rim area and cup size. Optic discs vary considerably in size, with the size of the optic disc cup correlating with the size of the optic disc.[2] In healthy individuals, a small disc will have a small cup, whereas a large disc will have a large cup (Figure 6-2). Therefore, large optic discs in healthy individuals tend to have large cups, which can lead to an erroneous

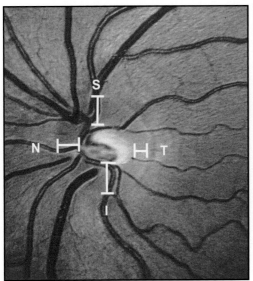

Figure 6-3. The configuration of the neuroretinal rim in a healthy eye generally follows the ISNT rule: the rim is usually widest **I**nferiorly, followed by **S**uperiorly, **N**asally, and, finally, **T**emporally.

diagnosis of glaucoma. On the other hand, small cups can be glaucomatous in small discs. There are several methods to evaluate optic disc size, including sophisticated imaging techniques. However, in clinical practice, the optic disc size can usually be estimated at the slit lamp with a high-magnification lens and by applying the appropriate correction factors.[3]

Step 2 relates to the evaluation of the neuroretinal rim. Identification of the neuroretinal rim width in all sectors of the optic disc is of fundamental importance for detecting diffuse and localized rim loss in glaucoma. The rim width should be measured as the distance between the border of the optic disc and the position of blood vessel bending. In healthy individuals, it is usually widest inferiorly, followed by superiorly, nasally, and, finally, temporally (ISNT rule; Figure 6-3).[4] Deviations from the ISNT rule should be noted, as well as areas of thinning or notching of the neuroretinal rim. Areas of neuroretinal rim loss can sometimes be identified by the presence of baring of the circumlinear vessel or bayoneting of vessels. During examination of the neuroretinal rim, the examiner should look for the presence of an acquired pit of the optic nerve as it is diagnostic of glaucoma and a sign usually associated with higher risk for progression.[1]

Step 3 describes the examination of the RNFL. The examiner should observe the brightness and striations of the RNFL as well as the visibility of the parapapillary vessels. Typically, these vessels are indistinct, but their borders become clearer as the RNFL is lost. RNFL loss can occur in a diffuse, localized, or mixed pattern. With diffuse loss, there is general reduction of the RNFL brightness, with reduction of the difference normally occurring between the superior and inferior poles compared with the temporal and nasal regions (Figure 6-4). Localized RNFL loss appears as wedge-shaped dark areas emanating from the optic disc in an arcuate pattern (Figure 6-5).[4]

Step 4 describes the examination of the parapapillary region, which is the area located just outside the optic disc. There are 2 forms of parapapillary atrophy (PPA): zone alpha (α) and zone beta (β). Zone α is present in most normal eyes as well as in eyes with glaucoma and is characterized by a region of irregular hypopigmentation and hyperpigmentation of the retinal pigment epithelium (RPE). The more important zone with respect to glaucoma is zone β, which is due to atrophy of the RPE and choriocapillaris, leading to increased visibility of the large choroidal vessels and sclera. Zone β is more common and extensive in eyes with glaucoma than in healthy eyes. The area of PPA is spatially correlated with the area of neuroretinal rim loss, with the atrophy being largest in the corresponding area of the thinner neuroretinal rim (Figure 6-6).[4]

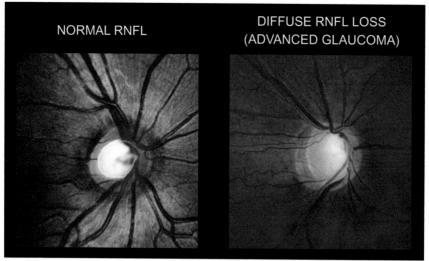

Figure 6-4. In patients with diffuse RNFL loss, there is a general reduction of the RNFL brightness and striations, with reduction of the difference normally existing between the superior and inferior poles compared with the temporal and nasal regions.

Figure 6-5. Localized RNFL loss appears as a wedge-shaped dark area emanating from the optic disc in an arcuate pattern.

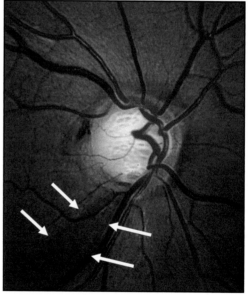

Step 5 refers to the active search for retinal and optic disc hemorrhages, which are suggestive of glaucoma progression (Figure 6-7).[5] Disc hemorrhages can be located over the neuroretinal rim, in the adjacent nerve fiber layer, or at the level of the lamina cribrosa. At times, they can be very small and may be missed unless meticulous examination is performed. They are transient, lasting from 2 to 6 months, but may recur.

As a final step, the examiner should compare the examination of one eye with that of the other eye, looking for the presence of asymmetry in the optic disc cup, which can be indicative of

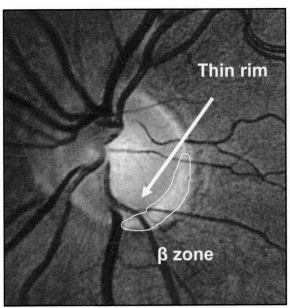

Figure 6-6. The area of zone β of PPA is spatially correlated with the area of neuroretinal rim loss, with the atrophy being largest in the corresponding area of thinner neuroretinal rim.

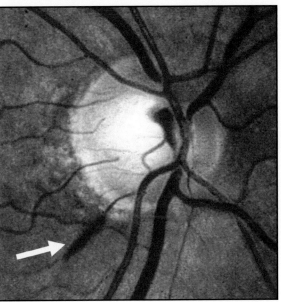

Figure 6-7. Flame-shaped hemorrhage (arrow) in the inferior temporal sector of the optic disc.

glaucomatous damage. It is noteworthy that, although some of the signs are more important than others, it is the combination of observations that will strengthen or weaken the diagnostic hypothesis of glaucoma.

Documentation of the appearance of the optic disc is as important as its examination. The appearance of the optic disc should be documented at baseline and during follow-up in all patients who have or are suspected of having glaucoma. Although fundamental, documentation of the optic disc appearance has been frequently neglected by clinicians. There are several methods available for optic disc documentation, including subjective (disc drawings) and objective (photographs and imaging methods) ones. Whenever available, an objective method should be used.

Optic disc photographs are still considered the gold standard for documentation and monitoring of optic disc appearance. Monocular photographs often fail to provide enough information on the contour of the optic disc cup to permit an adequate assessment of progressive changes, so whenever possible, stereophotographs should be used to document the optic disc appearance. Stereophotographs can be either simultaneous or nonsimultaneous (pseudo-stereophoto). Although simultaneous stereoscopic photographs are preferable, sequential pseudo-stereophotos are generally sufficient for adequate monitoring of the patient. If stereoscopic photographs are impossible to obtain, monocular photographs are still preferable to a simple schematic drawing or description of the appearance of the optic nerve.

Among the limitations of stereophotograph use for optic disc monitoring is the lack of consistency in the quality of photographs over time and the subjectivity involved in their interpretation. The comparison of photographs for detection of progression can be largely influenced by the examiner's skills. To reduce the subjectivity of optic disc evaluation, researchers have developed several objective imaging methods, such as confocal scanning laser ophthalmoscopy, scanning laser polarimetry, and optical coherence tomography (OCT).

References

1. Susanna R, Medeiros FA. *The Optic Nerve in Glaucoma*. 2nd ed. Rio de Janeiro, Brazil: Cultura Medica; 2006.
2. Britton RJ, Drance SM, Schulzer M, Douglas GR, Mawson DK. The area of the neuroretinal rim of the optic nerve in normal eyes. *Am J Ophthalmol*. 1987;103:497-504.
3. Garway-Heath DF, Rudnicka AR, Lowe T, Foster PJ, Fitzke FW, Hitchings RA. Measurement of optic disc size: equivalence of methods to correct for ocular magnification. *Br J Ophthalmol*. 1998;82:643-649.
4. Jonas JB, Budde WM, Panda-Jonas S. Ophthalmoscopic evaluation of the optic nerve head. *Surv Ophthalmol*. 1999;43:293-320.
5. Drance SM. Disc hemorrhages in the glaucomas. *Surv Ophthalmol*. 1989;33:331-337.

WHAT IMAGING TECHNOLOGY IS BEST FOR DIAGNOSING GLAUCOMA? FOR DETECTING PROGRESSION?

Christopher Leung, MD, MSc, BMedSc, MB ChB

Imaging Technologies for Evaluation of Glaucomatous Damage

Digital imaging is indispensable in providing objective and reproducible measurements of the optic nerve head and retinal nerve fiber layer (RNFL) for detection and monitoring of glaucoma. Confocal scanning laser ophthalmoscopy (CSLO), scanning laser polarimetry (SLP), and optical coherence tomography (OCT) are 3 prevailing imaging technologies for the evaluation of glaucomatous damage, with CSLO being the most long-standing and the spectral-domain OCT being the latest. These digital technologies differ in the principles of imaging and the parameters they can measure. While CSLO measures only optic disc parameters (eg, neuroretinal rim area, cup area, cup-to-disc ratios) and SLP measures only the circumpapillary RNFL thickness, OCT affords measurements of RNFL and optic disc parameters, as well as the inner macula thickness. All the imaging technologies have had significant improvements in the hardware and software configurations over the past decade. The latest generations of CSLO, SLP, and OCT are the HRT 3 (Heidelberg Retina Tomograph [HRT]; Heidelberg Engineering, GmbH, Heidelberg, Germany), GDx ECC (enhanced corneal compensation; Carl Zeiss Meditec, Dublin, California), and spectral-domain or Fourier-domain OCT (more than 6 different models have been introduced), respectively. The spectral-domain OCT has gained popularity in recent years for detecting glaucomatous damage and monitoring its progression due to its ability to image the optic disc and RNFL in high resolution.

Gedde SJ, ed. *Curbside Consultation in Glaucoma:*
49 Clinical Questions, Second Edition (pp 31–35)
© 2015 Taylor & Francis Group

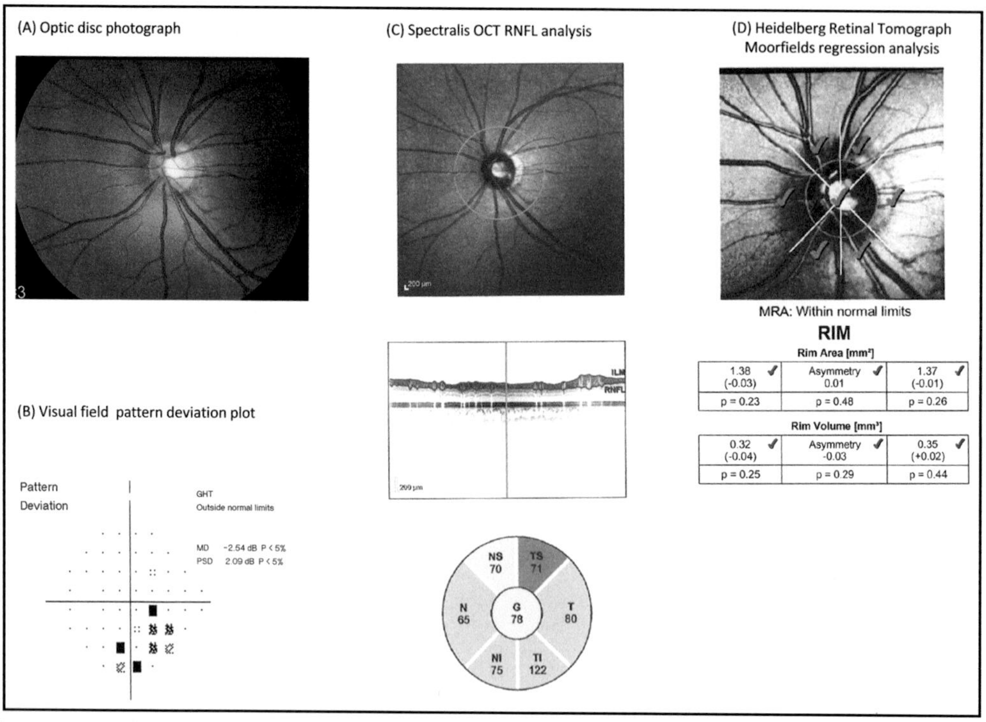

(A) Optic disc photograph

(C) Spectralis OCT RNFL analysis

(D) Heidelberg Retinal Tomograph Moorfields regression analysis

(B) Visual field pattern deviation plot

MRA: Within normal limits

RIM

Rim Area [mm²]

1.38 (-0.03) ✓	Asymmetry 0.01 ✓	1.37 (-0.01) ✓
p = 0.23	p = 0.48	p = 0.26

Rim Volume [mm³]

0.32 (-0.04) ✓	Asymmetry -0.03 ✓	0.35 (+0.02) ✓
p = 0.25	p = 0.29	p = 0.44

Pattern Deviation

GHT   Outside normal limits

MD   -2.54 dB P < 5%
PSD   2.09 dB P < 5%

Figure 7-1. A glaucomatous eye presented with an intraocular pressure (IOP) of 30 mm Hg and superior retinal nerve fiber layer (RNFL) thinning (A). Visual field examination revealed a corresponding inferonasal defect (mean deviation [MD] = −2.54, $P < .05$; PSD = 2.09 dB, $P < .05$; Glaucoma Hemifield Test—outside normal limits) (B). The Spectralis optical coherence tomograph (OCT) (Heidelberg Engineering GmbH, Heidelberg, Germany) confirmed the RNFL thinning at the superotemporal sector (C), although the Heidelberg Retinal Tomograph (HRT, Heidelberg Engineering) Moorfields regression analysis of the neuroretinal rim area was "within normal limits" (D). The RNFL thickness measured by the OCT was more sensitive to detect glaucomatous damage than the neuroretinal rim area measured by the HRT. (Adapted from Leung CK, Ye C, Weinreb RN, et al. Retinal nerve fiber layer imaging with spectral-domain optical coherence tomography: a study on diagnostic agreement with Heidelberg Retinal Tomograph. *Ophthalmology*. 2010;117:267-274.[2])

Detection of Glaucomatous Damage

Glaucomatous optic disc damage is characterized by progressive narrowing of the neuroretinal rim, cupping of the optic disc, and thinning of the RNFL. All imaging instruments have proprietary normative databases (ie, measurements obtained from normal healthy eyes) to classify whether the optic disc and RNFL measurements of an individual eye are within or outside the normal centile ranges. Because of the wide interindividual variations in optic disc size and neuroretinal rim configuration, the boundary between "normal" and "abnormal" neuroretinal rim measurement is often difficult to demarcate. For measurement of the neuroretinal rim area in CSLO, a reference plane (located 50 µm below the mean retinal surface outlined by a manually drawn contour line at the disc margin between 350 and 356 degrees) is adopted to delineate the neuroretinal rim (above the reference plane) and optic cup (below the reference plane). The arbitrary selection of the reference plane may render neuroretinal rim measurement less sensitive to signify glaucomatous damage (Figure 7-1). In fact, the neuroretinal rim area measured by the

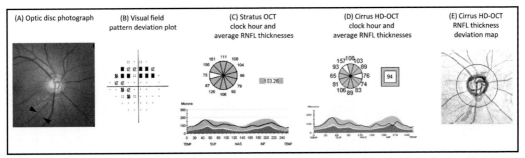

Figure 7-2. A glaucomatous eye with an inferotemporal RNFL defect barely visible in the fundus photograph (A) had superonasal defects in the visual field pattern deviation plot (B). While the Stratus OCT (Carl Zeiss Meditec, Dublin, California) (C) and the Cirrus HD-OCT (Carl Zeiss Meditec) (D) clock hour and average RNFL thicknesses failed to show any abnormality (all were within normal limits), the inferotemporal RNFL defect was evident in the RNFL thickness deviation map with abnormal pixels of RNFL measurement encoded in yellow and red. The RNFL thickness map is more informative to detect RNFL defects than the circumpapillary RNFL measurements. (Adapted from Leung CK, Lam S, Weinreb RN, et al. Retinal nerve fiber layer imaging with spectral-domain optical coherence tomography: analysis of the retinal nerve fiber layer map for glaucoma detection. *Ophthalmology.* 2010;117:1684-1691.[3])

CSLO has a lower sensitivity to detect glaucomatous damage compared with circumpapillary RNFL thickness measured by OCT or SLP at similar specificities.[1,2] While OCT RNFL and SLP RNFL measurements have comparable diagnostic performance for detection of glaucoma, the presence of atypical birefringence pattern in SLP has limited its application in eyes with hypopigmented fundus and myopia.

With the advent of spectral-domain OCT, it is feasible to perform a volumetric scan of the RNFL in the optic disc region and examine the patterns of RNFL defects in the RNFL thickness map. RNFL defects missed in the circumpapillary RNFL thickness profiles can be visualized in the RNFL thickness map (Figure 7-2), and the latter is more sensitive than the former to detect glaucomatous damage at a comparable level of specificity.[3] Collectively, the RNFL thickness map generated by the spectral-domain OCT is informative to determine the presence and the severity of optic nerve damage in patients with glaucoma. Of note, detection of RNFL thinning alone is not diagnostic of glaucoma. All optic neuropathies exhibit loss of retinal ganglion cells and nerve fibers. Biomicroscopic examination of the color and configuration of the neuroretinal rim is pertinent to differentiate glaucomatous from nonglaucomatous optic neuropathies.

Detection of Glaucoma Progression

Detection of glaucoma progression requires validated trend-based and/or event-based analyses.[4] Commercially available algorithms for progression analysis include the Topographic Change Analysis (TCA) in the HRT (Heidelberg Engineering) and the Guided Progression Analysis (GPA) in the GDx VCC/ECC (Carl Zeiss Meditec) and Cirrus HD-OCT (Carl Zeiss Meditec). TCA is an event-based analysis. It determines if there is significant elevation or depression in the surface height of the 15×15–degree optic nerve head region between the baseline and follow-up examinations (Figure 7-3A). GPA performs trend-based analyses (linear regression analysis) of the circumpapillary average and superior and inferior RNFL thicknesses, as well as event-based analyses of the circumpapillary RNFL thickness profile and the RNFL thickness maps (6×6 mm^2 for Cirrus HD-OCT and 20×20 degrees for GDx VCC/ECC, as shown in Figure 7-3B and 7-3C,

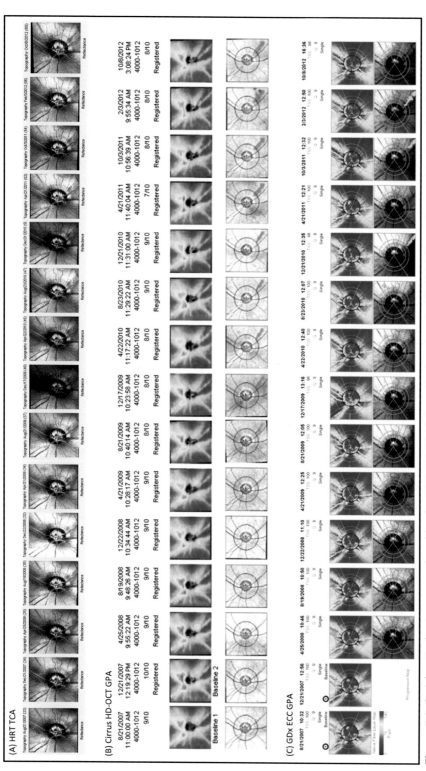

Figure 7-3. Serial optic disc images analyzed by the HRT TCA (Heidelberg Engineering GmbH, Heidelberg, Germany) (red pixels indicate significant surface depression and green pixels indicate significant surface elevation compared with the baseline examination) (A), and serial RNFL thickness maps (upper panel) and RNFL thickness change maps (lower panel) analyzed by the GPA in the Cirrus HD-OCT (Carl Zeiss Meditec, Dublin, California) (B) and the GDx ECC (Carl Zeiss Meditec) (C) of a glaucomatous eye (yellow pixels indicate significant reduction of RNFL thickness compared with baseline 1 and baseline 2, and red pixels indicate the reduction is confirmed in at least 2 consecutive follow-up visits). Progressive inferotemporal RNFL thinning was first confirmed in the OCT RNFL thickness change map on August 21, 2009, approximately 16 months before inferotemporal neuroretinal rim loss was evident in the HRT TCA on December 21, 2010, and approximately 37 months before RNFL retardance loss was confirmed in the GDx ECC GPA on October 8, 2012. It is notable that there is surface depression over the inferotemporal sector of the optic disc region in the HRT TCA on December 17, 2009, corresponding to the inferotemporal RNFL thinning detected by the Cirrus HD-OCT and GDx ECC GPA. (Adapted from Xu G, Weinreb RN, Leung CK. Retinal nerve fiber layer progression in glaucoma: a comparison between retinal nerve fiber layer thickness and retardance. *Ophthalmology.* 2013;120(12):2493-2500.[6])

respectively). While CSLO, SLP, and OCT have high reproducibility for measurements of the neuroretinal rim area and RNFL thickness, it is difficult to compare their performance for detection of glaucoma progression because the dynamic range of their measurements and the algorithms used for progression analysis vary considerably among the instruments. Measurement of progressive RNFL thinning may outperform measurement of progressive neuroretinal rim loss to detect eyes with glaucoma progression evident in optic disc stereophotography and standard automated perimetry.[5]

In theory, SLP may detect RNFL damage earlier than does OCT since disruption of the axonal microtubules (measured by SLP as a reduction in RNFL retardance) may precede loss of the nerve fiber bundles (measured by OCT as a reduction in RNFL thickness) in glaucoma. However, a prospective longitudinal study comparing the performance of GPA between GDx ECC and Cirrus HD-OCT showed that OCT detected progressive RNFL damage earlier than did SLP (Figure 7-3B and 7-3C).[6]

Summary

Analysis of the RNFL thickness map generated from the spectral-domain OCT is a promising approach to detect glaucomatous damage and monitor disease progression, although currently, most spectral-domain OCT systems are not equipped with the platform for RNFL thickness map analysis and progression analysis. It is worth noting that all imaging technologies are limited by the fact that they may not be sensitive enough to discern progressive optic disc and RNFL changes in the late stages of disease and that the detection of glaucoma is more complicated in myopic eyes, as the optic disc configuration and the distribution of RNFL bundles are different between myopes and nonmyopes.

References

1. Medeiros FA, Vizzeri G, Zangwill LM, Alencar LM, Sample PA, Weinreb RN. Comparison of retinal nerve fiber layer and optic disc imaging for diagnosing glaucoma in patients suspected of having the disease. *Ophthalmology.* 2008;115:1340-1346.
2. Leung CK, Ye C, Weinreb RN, et al. Retinal nerve fiber layer imaging with spectral-domain optical coherence tomography: a study on diagnostic agreement with Heidelberg Retinal Tomograph. *Ophthalmology.* 2010;117:267-274.
3. Leung CK, Lam S, Weinreb RN, et al. Retinal nerve fiber layer imaging with spectral-domain optical coherence tomography: analysis of the retinal nerve fiber layer map for glaucoma detection. *Ophthalmology.* 2010;117:1684-1691.
4. Weinreb RN, Garway-Heath D, Leung CK, Medeiros FA, Crowston JG, eds. *Consensus Series 8—Progression.* The Hague, the Netherlands: Kugler; 2011.
5. Alencar LM, Zangwill LM, Weinreb RN, et al. A comparison of rates of change in neuroretinal rim area and retinal nerve fiber layer thickness in progressive glaucoma. *Invest Ophthalmol Vis Sci.* 2010;51:3531-3539.
6. Xu G, Weinreb RN, Leung CK. Retinal nerve fiber layer progression in glaucoma: a comparison between retinal nerve fiber layer thickness and retardance. *Ophthalmology.* 2013;120(12):2493-2500.

WHAT VISUAL FIELD TESTS SHOULD I USE? HOW SHOULD I JUDGE PROGRESSION?

Angelo P. Tanna, MD and
Adam C. Breunig, MD

Visual field testing is critical in the diagnosis and management of glaucoma. The target intra-ocular pressure (IOP), the decision to initiate or intensify therapy, and the decision to advance to incisional surgery often hinge on the determination of the status of the visual field.

Visual Field Test Selection

The selection of a visual field testing strategy is based on the patient's visual acuity, the stage of the disease, and the location of the visual field damage. Achromatic, automated static perimetry or standard automated perimetry (SAP) is the most commonly used technique for visual field testing in the setting of glaucoma or suspicion of glaucoma. Although other testing approaches may ulti-mately prove to be superior for the early detection of glaucoma damage, SAP is the best technique to monitor patients over time for the detection of glaucoma progression.

In the past, full-threshold testing was the only available approach and often took 15 minutes per eye to complete. With advances in microprocessor speed, real-time calculations necessary to use advanced statistical modeling during the visual field test allow for the use of newer testing strategies such as Swedish interactive threshold algorithm (SITA) for the Humphrey perimeter and tendency-oriented perimetry (TOP) for the Octopus perimeter.

The SITA Standard testing algorithm allows for a higher degree of accuracy of the estimated threshold sensitivity values that are calculated compared with SITA Fast and is more reproducible, but it takes about 1 minute longer to perform per eye. For most purposes, we recommend the use of the SITA Standard testing algorithm. Most visual field damage in the setting of glaucoma can be detected using the 24-2 testing pattern in which the central 24 of the visual field are assessed along with 2 nasal locations that extend to 30 degrees from fixation. We recommend the use of the

Gedde SJ, ed. *Curbside Consultation in Glaucoma:*
49 Clinical Questions, Second Edition (pp 37–43)
© 2015 Taylor & Francis Group

24-2 SITA Standard testing strategy for most cases—this test typically takes about 5 minutes per eye.

Severe Damage

For eyes in which the field is severely damaged, the 10-2 pattern, which tests 68 locations spaced 2 degrees apart in the central 10 degrees of the visual field, often provides more useful information that can be tracked over time to determine if the disease is progressing (Figure 8-1). In addition, eyes with visual field damage near fixation should also be followed with 10-2 visual field tests. Progression sometimes can be detected in such eyes with the 10-2 testing algorithm, even though the 24-2 testing algorithm indicates stability. For eyes with substantial areas that are normal with the 24-2 test that also have paracentral visual field damage, we use both testing strategies and alternate them from visit to visit.

The default stimulus size for SAP is the Goldmann size III stimulus. Using the size V stimulus, which has a diameter 4 times larger, is useful in eyes with decreased visual acuity (20/50 or worse) or advanced glaucoma because it results in more reproducible results and allows for longer follow-up with computerized perimetry. SITA algorithms and normative data are unavailable for the size V stimulus; therefore, testing times are quite long, and computerized progression analysis is not readily available.

In eyes with very severe damage, SAP may no longer be helpful. In some such cases, Goldmann kinetic perimetry may yield useful results. Automated kinetic perimetry is now available using the Octopus perimeter.

Early Glaucoma

It has been demonstrated that some patients may lose a substantial number of retinal ganglion cells before SAP reveals the damage. This has generated interest in various perimetric techniques that may help improve sensitivity. Short-wavelength automated perimetry (SWAP) uses blue stimuli on a yellow background and preferentially tests retinal ganglion cells in the koniocellular pathway. Early studies suggested that it could detect glaucomatous visual field loss 3 to 5 years before standard automated perimetry; however, its superiority has been called into question in recent years.[1] We do not recommend the use of SWAP.

Frequency doubling technology (FDT) perimetry (FDT Matrix; Carl Zeiss Meditec, Irvine, California) may detect glaucomatous visual field damage earlier by preferentially stimulating retinal ganglion cells (RGCs) in the magnocellular pathway.[2]

Progression

One of the most challenging aspects of visual field analysis is determining whether progression has occurred. There is no reference standard for making this determination. Subjective evaluation of gray-scale maps of serial visual field tests is probably the most commonly used method, but this is usually not the best approach. In the course of visual field testing over time, a challenge the clinician faces in determining if progressive deterioration has occurred is the fact that the normal amount of fluctuation in visual sensitivity that occurs from test to test can mimic progressive glaucoma damage.

Computer-based strategies to help the clinician identify progression can be helpful. In general terms, 2 broad approaches are used: event-based methods and trend-based methods. Event-based methods define progression as having occurred once some predetermined degree of deterioration has taken place. Trend-based methods answer whether there is a statistically significant downward

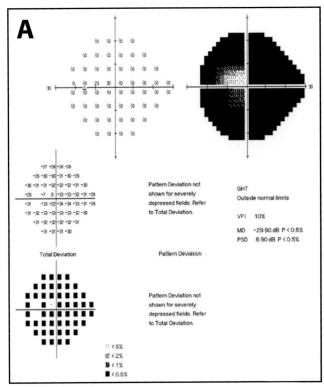

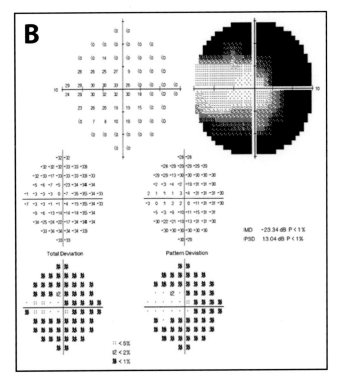

Figure 8-1. An example of a central island of remaining vision in a patient with advanced primary angle closure glaucoma. The 24-2 visual field test yields little useful information (A). The 10-2 test has locations within the central 10 degrees that are spaced 2 degrees apart (B), yielding more detailed information about the patient's visual function that can be monitored over time.

trend in some particular measure of the visual field, such as the mean deviation. These methods yield a rate of deterioration and a *P* value indicating the level of certainty the downward trend is real or due to chance alone.

Establishing a Baseline

In managing patients with glaucoma, an important early step the clinician must take is to establish a good set of baseline visual fields for future comparison. To do this, one must realize most patients must scale a learning curve before they are able to generate good-quality, reliable visual field tests that accurately depict their visual function. An abnormal visual field test, even if it meets reliability criteria and is consistent with other clinical findings, should be repeated to verify the characteristics of the abnormality. If the first 2 tests are reliable and look consistent, no further baseline testing is required. On the other hand, if the 2 tests yield substantially different results, as is often the case, the test should be repeated until you have a pair of similar, reliable tests. Later, if progression occurs and treatment is intensified, a new pair of reliable baseline visual field tests should be obtained.

Fluctuation in Threshold Sensitivity Measurements

When one tests the threshold sensitivity at a particular location in the visual field, one must anticipate a certain degree of variation or fluctuation from test to test. This is called *long-term fluctuation*. The magnitude of this fluctuation increases as a function of eccentricity (the further from fixation, the greater the variability) and severity of damage (the worse the damage at that location, the greater the variability). At some visits, the visual field will look a lot worse, even though the glaucoma is actually stable. Clinical trials have shown that even when deterioration of the visual field exceeds the 95% confidence interval of the expected degree of variation, one must repeat the test at least once, but preferably twice, to confirm the progression is real.

Event-Based Progression Analysis (Glaucoma Progression Analysis)

Glaucoma Progression Analysis (GPA; Carl Zeiss Meditec, Dublin, California) is the most important example of an event-based system. GPA uses essentially the same criteria used to define progression in the Early Manifest Glaucoma Trial (EMGT).[3] By performing repeat visual field testing 6 times over the course of about 1 month in approximately 100 stable patients with glaucoma, the EMGT investigators developed a database that was used to estimate the amount of expected fluctuation at a given location in the visual field at different levels of baseline damage severity.

The software defines the mean pattern deviation value of the first 2 visual field tests obtained as the baseline for each location (Figure 8-2). Each subsequent test result is compared with the baseline at each location. The database of stable patients with glaucoma described above is used to determine the 95% confidence interval of anticipated fluctuation as a function of testing location and damage severity. If a particular location has deteriorated more than this empirically determined magnitude of fluctuation, the location is marked by a triangle indicating significant deterioration (Figure 8-2B and 8-2C). If a particular location shows significant deterioration on 2 or at least 3 consecutive visual field tests, it is marked by a half-black or solid black triangle, respectively. If 3 or more locations are marked by half-black triangles, GPA identifies the visual field as showing "possible progression." If 3 or more locations are marked by solid black triangles, the visual field shows

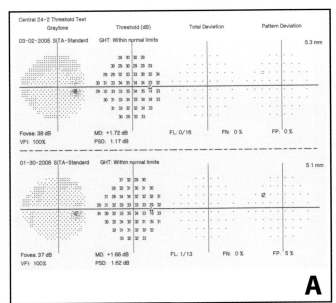

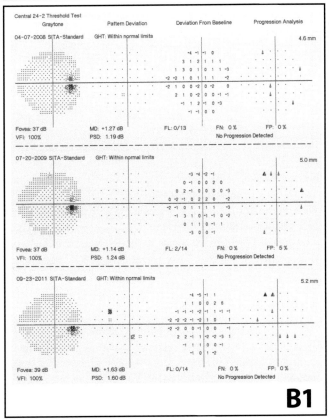

Figure 8-2. This patient presented with ocular hypertension in 2005, at which time he had a normal, reliable visual field. Because his estimated risk of conversion to primary open-angle glaucoma (POAG) was low, he elected observation without ocular hypotensive treatment. The first 2 baseline visual fields are normal (A). GPA uses the mean pattern deviation values from the first 2 fields for subsequent comparisons. The subsequent 3 visual field tests remain normal, and GPA classifies those as showing no progression (B1). The penultimate visual field test (B2) discloses several locations that are significantly worse than baseline. Because there are 3 locations with half-black or black triangles, the classification is "possible progression." In the EMGT, such a finding would have triggered repeat, confirmatory testing. In this case, the test was repeated within 2 months and the progression finding was verified. Because at least 3 locations have shown deterioration compared with baseline on 3 consecutive tests (solid black triangles), the test is classified as disclosing "likely progression" (B2). *(continued)*

Figure 8-2 (continued). This patient presented with ocular hypertension in 2005, at which time he had a normal, reliable visual field. Because his estimated risk of conversion to POAG was low, he elected observation without ocular hypotensive treatment. The visual field index (VFI) trend is downward sloping but not statistically significant (C). Small changes in the threshold sensitivity in the early stages of glaucoma often result in very small changes in the VFI. This example nicely illustrates the value of GPA and limitations of VFI trend analysis for the detection of glaucoma progression in the early stages of the disease.

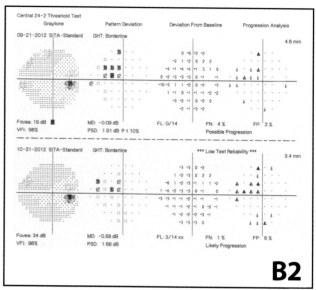

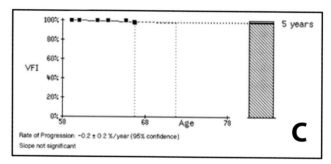

"likely progression" and would have met the EMGT criterion for progression. Of note, the locations marked by triangles need not be contiguous to signify progression.

A study comparing GPA analysis with the majority expert consensus by a group of glaucoma specialists found fair agreement, with GPA being more conservative in declaring progression compared with the experts.[4] The major limitations of GPA are its failure to detect progression when it occurs diffusely throughout much of the central 24 degrees of the visual field and its inability to detect progression in severe disease.

TREND-BASED PROGRESSION ANALYSIS

Examples of trend-based analyses include linear regression of the mean deviation (MD) or visual field index (VFI). Regression analysis of MD, for example, relates visual function to time by means of a straight-line equation but is limited because it does not distinguish between focal and diffuse change, either from glaucoma progression or media opacity. The VFI relies on both pattern deviation and total deviation data to express the severity of visual field damage as a percentage, with 100% being normal and 0% representing perimetric blindness. Linear regression analysis is performed on serial VFI values and can be used to calculate the rate of progression and a prediction of the future VFI if the previous trend continues.[5] Analysis of VFI trends is not useful for early glaucoma, primarily due to the small effect of early loss on global index values such as VFI; however, it often shows significant visual field progression when GPA fails to do so at later stages of the disease.

Progressive cataract causes deterioration in the visual field. The pattern deviation plot, GPA, and VFI are somewhat resistant to the impact of media opacity.

Clinicians may wonder, "Which type of analysis should be used and when?" In general, event- and trend-based analyses are complementary. Current GPA software incorporates the VFI trend analysis in its display. Event-based analysis may detect progression earlier, whereas trend-based methods may take longer to detect progression but are more useful in later stages of disease.

Even with advances in computer-aided interpretation, clinical judgment remains key in visual field interpretation. The entirety of the available clinical information should be used in clinical decision making. For cases in which the clinician is unsure about progression, repeat visual field testing is imperative.

References

1. Liu S, Lam S, Weinreb R, et al. Comparison of standard automated perimetry, frequency-doubling technology, and short-wavelength automated perimetry for detection of glaucoma. *Invest Ophthalmol Vis Sci.* 2011;52(10):7325-7331.
2. Medeiros FA, Sample PA, Weinreb RN. Frequency doubling technology perimetry abnormalities as predictors of glaucomatous visual field loss. *Am J Ophthalmol.* 2004;137:863-871.
3. Heijl A, Leske MC, Bengtsson B, Hussein M. Measuring visual field progression in the Early Manifest Glaucoma Trial. *Acta Ophthalmol Scand.* 2003;81:286-293.
4. Tanna AP, Budenz DL, Bandi JR, et al. Glaucoma progression analysis software compared with expert consensus opinion in the detection of visual field progression in glaucoma. *Ophthalmology.* 2012;119:468-473.
5. Bengtsson B, Heijl A. A visual field index for calculation of glaucoma rate of progression. *Arch Ophthalmol.* 2008;145:343-353.

WHAT ARE THE IMPLICATIONS OF DISC HEMORRHAGES IN GLAUCOMA PATIENTS OR SUSPECTS?

Jody R. Piltz-Seymour, MD

When you find a splinter hemorrhage on the optic disc, treat it as a warning signal that this eye is at risk for either developing glaucoma or for having progression of existing glaucomatous damage. Bjerrum first alluded to an association of optic disc hemorrhages (DHs) and glaucoma in 1889, but it was Drance and Begg[1] in 1970 who introduced DHs and their associated glaucoma risk into the modern literature. Since then, a myriad of reports have expounded on the relative risk of DHs for glaucoma, but many questions still remain.

DHs are often difficult to identify. While sometimes quite prominent, more often they are fine "splinter" linear hemorrhages that run radially along an often thinned area of the disc rim. At first glance, you may miss seeing the DH and mistake it for a blood vessel crossing the disc rim. When you look closer, however, you will notice that the linear red line of the DH does not extend over the retinal surface as a blood vessel would.

Identifying DHs clinically is difficult even for expert observers. In the Ocular Hypertension Treatment Study (OHTS), only 16% of photographically documented DHs were detected with dilated fundus examination.[2] Certainly, DHs can be more easily detected when trained readers are studying magnified disc photos, but it is important to remember that if you just look casually at the optic nerve, you will likely miss the majority of DHs. However, your ability to detect DHs will greatly increase if you leave time during each examination to carefully evaluate the optic disc.

DHs do not occur within a disc notch but rather will be found just at the edge of the notch (Figure 9-1). They develop most frequently on the inferior temporal rim, followed by the superior temporal rim. There is an increased incidence of β peripapillary atrophy and nerve fiber layer loss in the area of the DH. They are transient, persisting from 2 to 35 weeks, with a mean duration of 10.6 weeks. They may be recurrent and occasionally develop bilaterally, particularly in eyes with normal-tension glaucoma (NTG).[3]

Gedde SJ, ed. *Curbside Consultation in Glaucoma:*
49 Clinical Questions, Second Edition (pp 45–48)
© 2015 Taylor & Francis Group

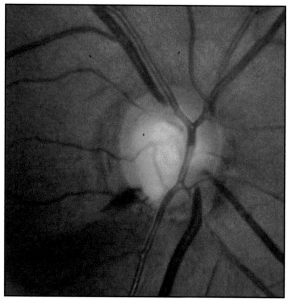

Figure 9-1. DH located at the edge of rim notch inferiorly. DHs occur most commonly inferiorly, at the edge of a notch and adjacent to a localized nerve fiber layer defect. β Peripapillary atrophy is also more prominent in the area of the DH.

DHs are uncommon in the healthy population and occur more frequently in glaucomatous eyes, especially those with NTG. The prevalence of DHs has been reported to be 5% to 25% in NTG, 2.4% to 8% in primary open-angle glaucoma (POAG), 1.5% to 5% in ocular hypertension (OHT), and 0% to 1.0% in normal eyes. The incidence of DH has been reported as 35.5% to 43% in NTG, 10.3% in POAG, and 10.4% in suspects during a follow-up of 3 to 13 years. Various studies have found an association between DHs and increasing age, female sex, large vertical cup-to-disc ratios, higher intraocular pressure (IOP), migraine headaches, type 2 diabetes mellitus, systemic hypertension, thinner corneas, and pseudoexfoliation.

The OHTS found that DHs were an independent risk factor for the development of glaucoma in eyes with OHT.[2] The risk of developing a POAG end point was 6 times more likely in patients with a DH. OHTS patients who developed DHs were older, had thinner corneas, and had larger baseline cup-to-disc ratios. The cumulative incidence of DH was 0.5% before the development of POAG and 2.5% per year in eyes after the development of POAG. Despite the increased rate of glaucoma, most OHTS patients with DH (87%) did not develop glaucoma, with mean follow-up of 31 months after the DH.

The evidence is very clear that DHs are a poor prognostic indicator. A recent study found that DH was the single most important predictor for visual field deterioration.[4] Disc hemorrhages may precede the development of localized notching and retinal nerve fiber layer (RNFL) defects (Figure 9-2). Studies have detected an increased incidence of progressive disc changes, nerve fiber layer loss, and visual field defects in glaucomatous eyes 1 to 5 years after the development of a DH (Figure 9-3). In the more recent OHTS report with a mean follow-up of 12 years, eyes with DH displayed visual field progression at more than twice the rate of eyes without DH. The increased risk of DH was found to be comparable to that of increasing age by 10.5 years, increasing IOP by 11 mm Hg, decreasing corneal thickness by 23 μm, or increasing the vertical cup-to-disc ratio by 0.1 unit.[5]

Does lowering IOP decrease the development of DHs? The answer is probably yes, but the evidence is not unequivocal. While the Early Manifest Glaucoma Trial (EMGT) did not find any difference in the presence or frequency of disc hemorrhages in treated and untreated eyes, the OHTS did.[6] With its large cohort of patients (2607 eyes of 1378 participants) and long follow-up

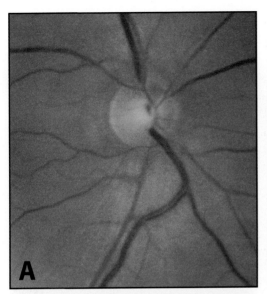

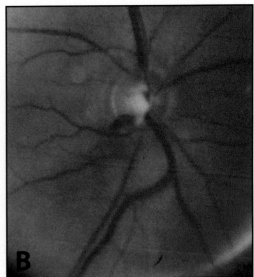

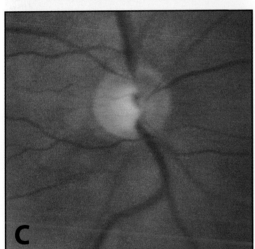

Figure 9-2. Progressive glaucomatous notching of the inferior optic disc rim at site of DH. (A) In 1992, the patient had an intact neuroretinal rim. The optic disc was small and no cupping was present, although the mild β peripapillary atrophy was a risk factor for future glaucoma in this patient. (B) Notching with an adjacent DH was noted in 1996. (C) The notch extended after this episode, as documented in the 2001 photograph.

(mean [SD] of 12 [2] years), OHTS reported that IOP lowering significantly reduced the risk of developing DHs.[5] In addition, a surgical trial also noted a marked decrease in the rate of development of DHs after trabeculectomy in both POAG and NTG groups.[7]

While DHs are strongly associated with glaucoma, they are not specific to glaucoma. Occasionally, DHs may develop in association with other ocular disorders such as posterior vitreous detachments, retinal vascular occlusive disease, optic disc drusen, and nonglaucomatous optic neuropathies or with systemic disorders such as systemic hypertension, type 2 diabetes mellitus, leukemia, or systemic lupus erythematosus.

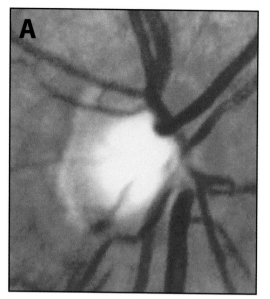 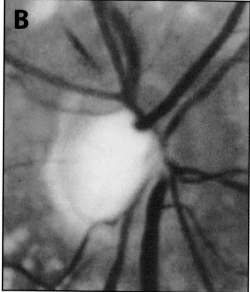

Figure 9-3. This is another example of progressive cupping at the site of a prior DH. (A) DH present inferiorly. (B) There is loss of the inferior rim at the site of the prior hemorrhage. Also note the presence of a superior splinter hemorrhage adjacent to the disc edge superiorly. It is easy to overlook these thin, linear splinter hemorrhages.

Summary

It is very important to closely examine the optic disc in search of DHs. While not all hemorrhages lead to ongoing glaucomatous loss, it is important to consider the presence of a DH as a significant risk factor for the development or progression of glaucomatous optic nerve, nerve fiber layer, and visual field loss. You need to follow these patients more closely and consider more aggressive management to decrease the risk of progressive glaucomatous damage.

References

1. Drance SM, Begg IS. Sector hemorrhage: a probable acute ischemic disc change in chronic simple glaucoma. *Can J Ophthalmol.* 1970;5:137-141.
2. Budenz DL, Anderson DR, Feuer WJ, et al. Detection and prognostic significance of optic disc hemorrhages during the Ocular Hypertension Treatment Study. *Ophthalmology.* 2006;113:2137-2143.
3. Gordon J, Piltz-Seymour JR. The significance of optic disc hemorrhages in glaucoma. *J Glaucoma.* 1997;6:62-64.
4. De Moraes CG, Liebmann JM, Park SC et al. Optic disc progression and rates of visual field change in treated glaucoma. *Acta Ophthalmol.* 2013;91:e86-e91.
5. De Moraes CG, Demirel S, Gardiner SK, et al. Rate of visual field progression in eyes with optic disc hemorrhages in the Ocular Hypertension Treatment Study. *Arch Ophthalmol.* 2012;130(12):1541-1546.
6. Bengtsson B, Leske MC, Yang Z, Heijl A. Disc hemorrhages and treatment in the Early Manifest Glaucoma Trial. *Ophthalmology.* 2008;115:2044-2048.
7. Miyake T, Sawada A, Yamamoto T, et al. Incidence of disc hemorrhages in open-angle glaucoma before and after trabeculectomy. *J Glaucoma.* 2006;15:164-171.

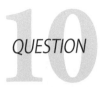

How Should I Follow Patients With Anomalous Optic Discs, Such as Those With Optic Nerve Drusen, Tilted Discs, Myopic Discs, and Discs With Pits?

Jane Loman, MD and
Joseph Caprioli, MD

Anomalous optic discs can make the evaluation for and of glaucoma difficult. Typical characteristics of the optic nerve, such as a well-defined disc margin or a distinct cup-to-disc ratio, may not be present. Anomalous nerves may also be associated with atypical visual field (VF) defects but are also not immune to glaucomatous damage. Thus, the clinician must recognize other key features of glaucomatous nerves, as well as the different patterns of VF loss in patients with glaucoma, tilted discs, myopic discs, and discs with drusen and pits. Even if glaucoma is initially ruled out, many of these patients should be monitored as glaucoma suspects, with serial optic disc photos and VF tests. Changes should prompt reevaluation for glaucoma or other abnormalities associated with anomalous discs. Optical coherence topography (OCT), confocal scanning laser ophthalmoscopy, or scanning laser polarimetry has not proven to be consistently useful to monitor atypical discs. To counsel these patients, it is important to know the prevalence, natural history, clinical features, treatment, proposed pathophysiology, and complications of these diseases.

Optic Nerve Drusen

The overall prevalence of optic nerve drusen (OND) is around 0.4% to 2%. OND may be congenital, be inherited in an autosomal-dominant fashion, and become more clinically apparent with age. It is thought that this is a disorder of axoplasmic flow that leads to drusen formation that can damage the nerve fiber layer (NFL) or vascular structures.[1] Patients may present with symptoms of transient visual obscurations, but OND is often an incidental finding. Signs of OND range between visible and buried drusen. Calcified buried drusen can be diagnosed with B-scan ultrasound, autofluorescence on fluorescein angiography, or computed tomography. On examination, OND disc margins are obscured, and the vessels are tortuous with central branching and can

Gedde SJ, ed. *Curbside Consultation in Glaucoma:*
49 Clinical Questions, Second Edition (pp 49–54)
© 2015 Taylor & Francis Group

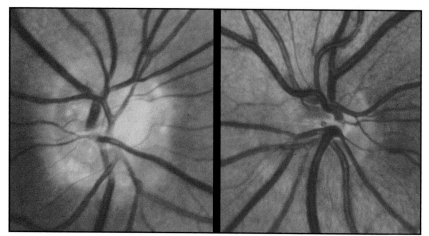

Figure 10-1. OND, both eyes (OU): There are some visible drusen, right eye (OD) and buried drusen, left eye (OS) with associated obscured disc margins.

Figure 10-2. Optic nerve drusen OD: inferior nerve fiber layer loss causing corresponding visual defect and OCT findings.

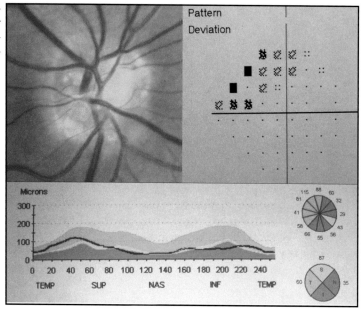

consist of many cilioretinal arteries. There is often no physiologic cup (Figure 10-1). Upon initial examination, efforts must be made to find the rim of the disc that may show thinning and suggest concomitant optic nerve damage. Other key features are NFL defects from glaucoma or from the compressive effects of a druse itself. These may be more noticeable with red-free disc photos. In select patients, OCT may be a useful tool for following the NFL if it also correlates with clinical examination and VF testing (Figure 10-2).[1,2] Seventy percent to 90% of patients present with very early VF defects (enlarged blind spots, general constriction, or glaucoma-like nasal steps and arcuate scotomas) that may progress slowly at a rate of 1.6% in one study or not at all. Other rare complications of this disease include anterior ischemic optic neuropathy (3%) and choroidal neovascularization (CNV). Thus far, there is no proven treatment for this disease, but most patients will retain good vision and should be observed with serial VF tests and optic disc photos.

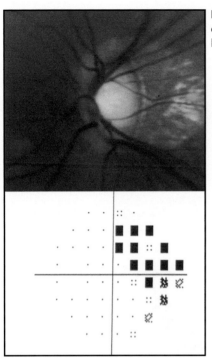

Figure 10-3. Tilted disc: this tilted disc is associated with a VF defect that has not changed in 3 years of follow-up. The patient has received no treatment.

Intraocular pressure (IOP) lowering has been suggested for patients who have glaucomatous VF defects or NFL loss, even though it is difficult to differentiate NFL loss from glaucoma or the compressive effects of the drusen themselves.

Tilted Disc Syndrome

The prevalence of tilted disc syndrome (TDS) is approximately 1.6%.[3] This syndrome must be differentiated from the common occurrence of a nontorsional temporally tilted disc that can have nonprogressing VF changes (Figure 10-3). TDS is a congenital syndrome that results from defective embryonic fissure closure. In the Blue Mountain Eye Study, it was defined as having inferior or nasal tilting of the disc that tended to be associated with the following signs: inferonasal torsion of the disk, refractive astigmatism with mild myopia, situs inversus of the retinal vessels, β peripapillary atrophy (β-PPA), inferonasal chorioretinal thinning, and posterior staphyloma or coloboma (Figure 10-4).[3] The tilted disc rim can result in the superotemporal elevation of the NFL and blur the disc margin, which can be confused with disc swelling or buried drusen. These patients occasionally present with atypical VF defects mimicking bitemporal hemianopia. They are differentiated from chiasmal lesions because the defects are stable, are less dense, and cross the vertical meridian. More serious complications of this disease include macular detachment, atrophy, and CNV that are easily differentiated with OCT. The combination of β-PPA, VF defects, and a difficult-to-interpret disc may lead clinicians to suspect glaucoma, but recognizing the other characteristic signs and complications of TDS should preclude a misdiagnosis of glaucoma. These patients should be examined regularly for macular involvement, VF changes, and ocular hypertension.

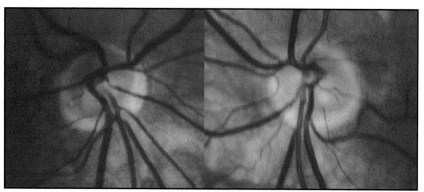

Figure 10-4. TDS OU: inferonasal torsion of right and left discs.

Myopic Discs

In population-based studies, the prevalence of myopia and glaucoma is 4% and may increase to 6% to 7% with higher degrees of myopia. This increased prevalence compared with nonmyopic patients (1% to 2%) is not confirmed in randomized controlled studies.[4] It is thought that these patients may have a thinner lamina cribrosa that is subject to scleral wall stress and may be associated with a thinner cornea. Some optic nerves may have a focal weakness in their architecture, and IOP-related problems may spare other areas of the disc. These discs have oval shapes, large regions of β-PPA, and shallow diffuse cupping. They are typically tilted temporally, which may obscure both the temporal and nasal rims. The inferior and superior rims should still be interpretable and are important in glaucoma evaluation (Figure 10-5).[5] Visual field analysis may show arcuate scotomas that correspond to thin or nonexistent rim tissue at the inferior and superior poles. Atypical or central VF scotomas may be due to myopic degeneration (Figure 10-6). Glaucoma treatment is often started in patients with identifiable thinning of the rim and VF defect; however, when the pretreatment IOP is already low, it may be prudent to find definitive signs of progression before instating more aggressive treatment, especially since the optic nerve abnormality may be focal and stable. These patients are also at higher risk for hypotony maculopathy after surgery.[5]

Congenital and Acquired Optic Pits

The prevalence of congenital optic pits (COPs) is <1% and must be differentiated from acquired optic pits (AOPs) that are due to focal glaucomatous damage. A COP results from malclosure of the embryonic fissure and is usually an incidental finding (Figure 10-7). It is a temporal focal depression of the optic disc that may produce VF defects by displacing focal areas of NFL. The pit typically does not affect the superior and inferior poles, and thus glaucoma evaluation should not be difficult. The most common complications of COPs are serous macular detachments and schisis, which eventually occur in 40% of these patients and can be demonstrated on OCT. In contrast, AOPs have a prevalence rate of 5% to 9% within a group of patients with glaucoma.[6] The pathophysiology of AOPs is unknown but occurs most often in patients with normal-tension glaucoma who have recurrent disc hemorrhages. It is defined as a localized deep excavation of the neural rim with focal loss of normal laminar architecture.[7] The region is pale with no rim tissue remaining next to the disc edge (Figure 10-8). Paracentral VF defects are more common in patients with glaucoma who do not have AOPs. The existence of an AOP is a risk factor for glaucoma progression.[6] Thus, these patients should be followed closely with VF tests and serial optic disc photos.

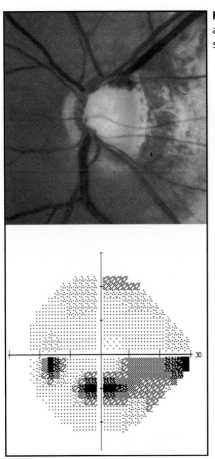

Figure 10-5. Myopic disc (–10 D) and glaucoma: myopic disc and glaucomatous optic nerve damage with disc hemorrhage superiorly.

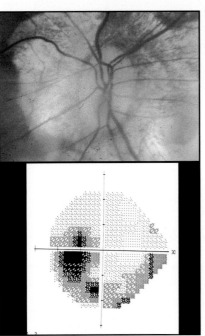

Figure 10-6. Myopic degeneration (–17 D): myopic disc with myopic fundus changes accounting for an atypical VF. There have been no changes in VF in the past 4 years.

Figure 10-7. Congenital optic nerve pit: temporal optic nerve pit with a normal VF.

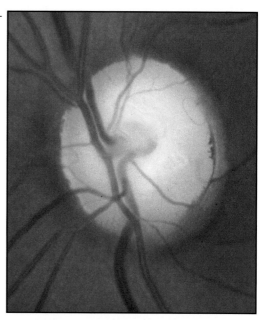

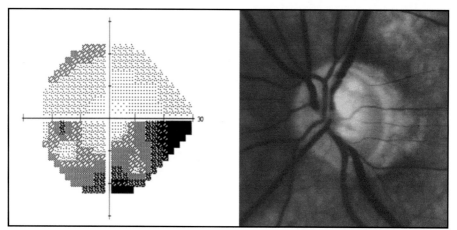

Figure 10-8. Acquired optic nerve pit: focal glaucomatous optic nerve damage with corresponding inferior arcuate.

References

1. Davis PL, Jay WM. Optic nerve head drusen. *Semin Ophthalmol.* 2003;18:222-242.
2. Katz BJ, Pomeranz HD. Visual field defects and retinal nerve fiber layer defects in eyes with buried optic nerve drusen. *Am J Ophthalmol.* 2006;141:248-253.
3. Vongphanit J, Mitchell P, Wang JJ. Population prevalence of tilted optic disks and the relationship of this sign to refractive error. *Am J Ophthalmol.* 2002;133:679-685.
4. Xu L, Wang Y, Wang S, Jonas JB. High myopia and glaucoma susceptibility: the Beijing Eye Study. *Ophthalmology.* 2007;114:216-220.
5. Burgoyne C. Myopic eyes and glaucoma. *J Glaucoma.* 2004;13:85-86.
6. Ugurlu S, Weitzman M, Nduaguba C, Caprioli J. Acquired pit of the optic nerve: a risk factor for progression of glaucoma. *Am J Ophthalmol.* 1998;125:457-464.
7. Spaeth GL. A new classification of glaucoma including focal glaucoma. *Surv Ophthalmol.* 1994;38(suppl):S9-S17.

HOW FREQUENTLY SHOULD I PERFORM FOLLOW-UP EXAMINATIONS, GONIOSCOPY, VISUAL FIELD TESTING, AND OPTIC NERVE EVALUATION IN PATIENTS WITH GLAUCOMA?

Dana M. Blumberg, MD, MPH; Paul P. Lee, MD, JD;
and Reena S. Vaswani, MD

Primary open-angle glaucoma (POAG) is a chronic optic neuropathy diagnosed by characteristic optic nerve and/or visual field abnormalities. Traditionally, elevated intraocular pressure (IOP) of 21 mm Hg or greater was required for glaucoma diagnosis; however, it is no longer necessary as up to half of those with POAG have normal IOP measurements.[1] Thus, examining the optic disc is the most important initial diagnostic step, ideally using appropriate magnification, illumination, and binocular viewing (typically an indirect lens from 78 to 90 D in a dilated eye). Clinical examination of the optic nerve should focus on detecting characteristic structural changes, including generalized or focal enlargement of the optic cup, thinning of the neuroretinal rim, disc hemorrhages, peripapillary atrophy, and thinning of the nerve fiber layer. The assessment should be documented with color stereophotography, computer-based imaging analysis, or at least a detailed drawing or description.

To supplement structural assessment, functional evaluation of the visual field (VF)—most commonly automated static perimetry—indicates the degree of measurable vision compromise. It is important to ensure that the test is reliable and that the visual field damage is consistent with the presumed underlying pathology. The visual field defect should correlate with glaucomatous changes in the optic nerve head, and lack of such correlation should raise concern about other etiologies for the visual field damage. Initial visual fields often need to be repeated for suspected defects to determine whether they are artifactual or true documentation of disease. Clinical trials have demonstrated that as many as 88% of initial glaucomatous visual field defects are not validated on repeat testing.[2] Thus, an abnormal baseline VF should be repeated, usually within a 3 to 6 month interval.

Assessing whether the nerve has been damaged as a result of POAG vs primary angle closure glaucoma requires skilled gonioscopy. If the pigmented trabecular meshwork cannot be visualized, the patient is at risk for POAG, and a prophylactic peripheral iridotomy should be considered. In

Gedde SJ, ed. *Curbside Consultation in Glaucoma:*
49 Clinical Questions, Second Edition (pp 55–57)
© 2015 Taylor & Francis Group

addition, gonioscopy can identify secondary mechanisms of elevated eye pressure such as pigment dispersion, pseudoexfoliation, angle recession and traumatic angle damage, neovascularization resulting from ischemia, and peripheral anterior synechiae from inflammation. It is important that we periodically reevaluate patients at risk for angle closure annually and once every 5 years for those at lower risk or upon the initiation of medications that may alter the angle configuration.

Once the diagnosis of POAG is made, we should discuss the merits of treatment with the patient. Several large-scale clinical trials, which have included different stages of disease, have given us insight into the necessary IOP reduction from baseline to reduce the rate of worsening of glaucomatous disease.[3–8] Across these studies, the greater the degree of IOP reduction, the lower the rate of worsening has been found. Establishment of an individualized target pressure range, based on the level of damage and, if possible, the IOP at which this damage has occurred, helps guide therapy. For those uncomfortable with target pressure determination, a usable rule of thumb for determining the initial target pressure is to lower the IOP 20% to 30%[1,2] from the pretreatment value, with IOPs consistently below 18 mm Hg.[9] The important point to remember about target pressure is that we cannot definitively state what the target pressure should be; instead, we should use it as a yardstick with which to measure the effects of our treatment. If a patient has not achieved target pressure, we should modify treatment until our goal IOP is reached. If, however, target IOP is still not achieved, we should consider the pros and cons of adding additional treatment vs the risk of glaucoma progression. Some clinicians wait for a sign of progression (ie, elevated IOP *and* structural and/or functional changes before adding treatment), whereas others may adjust treatment based on elevated IOP alone. In certain circumstances, increasing the target pressure upward may be justified.

The degree or stage of glaucoma damage can be categorized with one of several systems; the American Academy of Ophthalmology (AAO) Preferred Practice Pattern uses 3 broad categories (mild, moderate, and severe) based on visual field loss. Findings from Olmsted County confirm prior studies demonstrating that those with severe visual field loss at presentation are significantly more likely to become blind during their lifetimes. Thus, more aggressive therapy and follow-up are indicated for those with more severe visual field loss. Patients whose IOP exceeds the target pressure or who have shown recent progression of the nerve or VF should have more aggressive treatment and more frequent follow-up. Follow-up visits may need to be performed within 4 months, and optic nerve evaluations and visual fields may be performed at each of these visits. Alternatively, patients who have more moderate stable glaucoma and well-controlled IOP may need only a follow-up visit, optic nerve examination, and visual field testing twice a year. Patients with well-controlled mild glaucoma or glaucoma suspects may be monitored with a semiannual examination with an annual visual field and optic nerve head examination.

Recent evidence suggests that clinical practice may not always be consistent with these guidelines.[9] In one study, only 53% of patients with glaucoma had an annual optic nerve photograph or drawing, and 43% of those with moderate to severe glaucoma had visual field tests less than once a year.[10] Furthermore, IOP was uncontrolled in nearly half of follow-up visits in patients with moderate to severe glaucoma. Recent data indicate that, on average, patients receive less than one VF per year and are examined approximately every 8 months, regardless of disease severity or visual field progression.[11] Over the past decade, visual field utilization has been shown to decrease while use of optic nerve imaging has proportionally increased. Since ophthalmic imaging has not yet been proven to be as effective in detecting glaucomatous progression as visual field, these practices may be detrimental to patient care.[12] Higher levels of provider adherence to published guidelines will likely result in decreased visual loss from glaucoma. Since most patients with glaucoma will not subjectively notice signs of deterioration, it is incumbent on us to monitor all patients with glaucoma with appropriate diagnostic testing and therapeutic interventions.

References

1. Sommer A, Tielsch JM, Katz J, et al. Relationship between intraocular pressure and primary open angle glaucoma among Black and White Americans: the Baltimore Eye Study. *Arch Ophthalmol.* 1991;109:1090.
2. Keltner JL, Johnson CA, Spurr JO, Kass MA, Gordon MO; the OHTS Group. Confirmation of visual field abnormalities in the ocular hypertension treatment study. *Invest Ophthalmol Vis Sci.* 1998;39:S493.
3. Collaborative Normal-Tension Glaucoma Study Group. Comparison of glaucomatous progression between untreated patients with normal-tension glaucoma and patients with therapeutically reduced intraocular pressures. *Am J Ophthalmol.* 1998;126:487-497.
4. Collaborative Normal-Tension Glaucoma Study Group. The effectiveness of intraocular pressure reduction in the treatment of normal-tension glaucoma. *Am J Ophthalmol.* 1998;126:498-505.
5. Gordon MO, Beiser JA, Brandt JD, et al. The Ocular Hypertension Treatment Study: baseline factors that predict the onset of primary open-angle glaucoma. *Arch Ophthalmol.* 2002;120:714-720, discussion 829-830.
6. Heijl A, Leske MC, Bengtsson B, et al. Reduction of intraocular pressure and glaucoma progression: results from the Early Manifest Glaucoma Trial. *Arch Ophthalmol.* 2002;120:1268-1279.
7. Leske MC, Heijl A, Hussein M, et al. Factors for glaucoma progression and the effect of treatment: the Early Manifest Glaucoma Trial. *Arch Ophthalmol.* 2003;121:48-56.
8. The AGIS Investigators. The Advanced Glaucoma Intervention Study (AGIS), 7: the relationship between control of intraocular pressure and visual field deterioration. The AGIS Investigators. *Am J Ophthalmol.* 2000;130:429-440.
9. Hertzog LH, Albrecht KG, LaBree L, Lee PP. Glaucoma care and conformance with preferred practice patterns: examination of the private, community-based ophthalmologist. *Ophthalmology.* 1996;103:1009-1013.
10. Fremont AM, Lee PP, Mangione CM, et al. Patterns of care for open-angle glaucoma in managed care. *Arch Ophthalmol.* 2003;121:777-783.
11. Fung SM, Lerner C, Russell RA, et al. Are practical recommendations practiced? A national multi-center cross sectional study on frequency of visual field testing in glaucoma. *Br J Ophthalmol.* 2013;97:843-847.
12. Stein J, Talwar N, Laverne A, et al. Trends in utilization of ancillary glaucoma tests for patients with open angle glaucoma from 2001 to 2009. *Ophthalmology.* 2012;119(4):748-758.

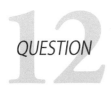

SHOULD I MEASURE CENTRAL CORNEAL THICKNESS IN ALL PATIENTS WITH GLAUCOMA? ALL GLAUCOMA SUSPECTS?

James D. Brandt, MD

In 2002, the Ocular Hypertension Treatment Study (OHTS) reported that central corneal thickness (CCT) was a powerful predictive factor for the development of glaucoma.[1] This finding was externally verified by the European Glaucoma Prevention Study (EGPS), and CCT plays an important role in the merged OHTS/EGPS risk model,[2] available online at http://ohts.wustl.edu /risk/calculator.html.

Confronted with the expanding evidence that CCT is an important ocular parameter that should be measured, most clinicians acquire pachymetry measurements in their patients but then wonder what to do with the information.

Risk Factor or Tonometry Artifact?

The OHTS investigators were careful to call CCT a "predictive" rather than a "risk" factor.[1] The difference is more than semantics—the term *risk factor* implies an environmental or biological link to disease causation, whereas *predictive factor* simply describes an association between something that can be measured and a later disease-associated event. In models like the one generated by the OHTS, the reported hazard ratio represents the increased (or decreased) risk of an outcome (in OHTS, the development of a glaucomatous end point) associated with a difference in a baseline measurement compared with the average for the population studied. The average CCT in the OHTS was 572.5 µM; a hazard ratio of 1.71 was found for CCTs 40 µM thinner than this average. In other words, an individual with a CCT of 532.5 µM had a 71% greater risk of developing glaucoma than the average OHTS participant.

A predictive model tells us nothing about causation. When the pachymetry protocol was added to the OHTS,[3] most of the investigators (myself included) believed that the impact of CCT in the

Gedde SJ, ed. *Curbside Consultation in Glaucoma:
49 Clinical Questions, Second Edition* (pp 59–61)
© 2015 Taylor & Francis Group

OHTS would be primarily through the effect of CCT as an artifact of Goldmann applanation tonometry (GAT) measurements. A variety of correction nomograms have been proposed to adjust intraocular pressure (IOP) based on CCT. Based on limited numbers of patients, these nomograms are useful when exploring data from groups of patients but are not valid in individual patients. It is notable that attempts to model and adjust the OHTS IOP data using every published correction nomogram for GAT and CCT have thus far failed to eliminate CCT as a predictive factor from the OHTS multivariate model,[4] suggesting that there may in fact be a biological link between CCT and glaucoma pathophysiology.

Adjusting Intraocular Pressure Is not Useful in Daily Practice

The enthusiasm with which clinicians embraced pachymetry reflected the belief that they would then be able to adjust GAT measurements in individual patients to arrive at a more accurate estimate of IOP. Unfortunately, this approach confuses accuracy (how close a measurement is to the true value) with precision (the repeatability of a measurement). Clinicians often fail to appreciate the significant imprecision of the Goldmann tonometer in most clinical settings—in even the most rigorous settings (eg, an IOP-focused clinical trial), GAT precision is approximately ± 2.5 mm Hg.[5] Compounding this inherent imprecision is the fact that many tonometers in clinical use are out of calibration, and few clinicians carry out calibration checks of their tonometers on a regular basis.[6]

The only way to arrive at an accurate estimate with a relatively imprecise device like the Goldmann tonometer is to take multiple measurements and average the results—the more measurements one acquires, the more likely the average approaches the true value (assuming no bias of the underlying technique—this is where CCT and other aspects of corneal biomechanics come into play). Thus, applying a "correction" to a single, imprecise measurement does not lead to a more accurate result.

Should I Measure CCT in Everyone? How Should I Use the Information?

Despite the shift in focus from IOP to the optic nerve in our working definition of glaucoma, elevated IOP is often the first signal to a clinician to look for the disease. In my opinion, clinicians should simply measure CCT in everyone—it only takes a few seconds per eye but can pay dividends in disease detection. As more patients undergo corneal refractive surgery, a growing proportion will have artificially lowered IOP measurements. In a few years, most will forget to tell their doctor about their LASIK or photorefractive keratectomy (PRK) they had in their youth. We have all seen patients whose glaucoma was detected in an advanced stage because tonometry was "normal" after PRK in the 1980s. This problem will only grow.

If there is no validated correction algorithm for adjusting IOP in an individual patient, but CCT demonstrably affects glaucoma risk, how should the clinician use CCT in daily practice? If there is one thing I have learned over the past decade of performing pachymetry is that just as it is important to recognize that optic discs come in small, medium, and large (allowing the clinician to interpret cup-to-disc ratios in context), one can take far better care of patients simply by categorizing corneas as thin, average, or thick. I have come to define *average* in my practice as being between 520 and 580 μm and view IOP measurements in patients with CCTs outside this range with an extra dose of skepticism. Trying to be more specific than this is simply not feasible.

Measuring CCT leads to the discontinuation of therapy in many overtreated ocular hypertensives and escalation of therapy in patients with thin corneas in whom control is clearly inadequate. Adding pachymetry to the decision making in patients with ocular hypertension and glaucoma helps refine which patients need further attention and who can be considered at low risk of developing damage.[7] Ultimately, incorporating the measurement of CCT into the glaucoma examination allows the astute clinician to better target and titrate his or her surveillance and treatment of glaucoma.

References

1. Gordon MO, Beiser JA, Brandt JD, et al. The Ocular Hypertension Treatment Study: baseline factors that predict the onset of primary open-angle glaucoma. *Arch Ophthalmol.* 2002;120:714-720.
2. Ocular Hypertension Treatment Study Group, European Glaucoma Prevention Study Group, Gordon MO, et al. Validated prediction model for the development of primary open-angle glaucoma in individuals with ocular hypertension. *Ophthalmology.* 2007;114:10-19.
3. Brandt JD, Beiser JA, Kass MA, Gordon MO. Central corneal thickness in the Ocular Hypertension Treatment Study (OHTS). *Ophthalmology.* 2001;108:1779-1788.
4. Brandt JD, Gordon MO, Gao F, et al. Adjusting intraocular pressure for central corneal thickness does not improve prediction models for primary open-angle glaucoma. *Ophthalmology.* 2012;119:437-442.
5. Tonnu PA, Ho T, Sharma K, et al. A comparison of four methods of tonometry: method agreement and interobserver variability. *Br J Ophthalmol.* 2005;89:847-850.
6. Kumar N, Hillier RJ. Goldmann tonometer calibration: a national survey. *Eye (Lond).* 2009;23:413-415.
7. Sandhu J, Pushpoth S, Birch M, Ray-Chaudhuri N. The role of pachymetry in primary care as a refinement tool of ocular hypertension and glaucoma referrals. *Br J Ophthalmol.* 2011;95:1758.

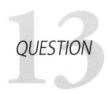

WHAT NEW METHODS ARE AVAILABLE TO MEASURE INTRAOCULAR PRESSURE? ARE ANY DEVICES AVAILABLE FOR CONTINUOUS MONITORING OF INTRAOCULAR PRESSURE?

Arthur J. Sit, MD, SM

Intraocular Pressure Measurement in the Clinic

Measurement of intraocular pressure (IOP) is a remarkably complex process in clinical patients. This stems from the fact that true pressure measurement can only be accomplished through manometry, during which the eye is cannulated, and the cannula is connected to a manometer (such as a water column or any type of calibrated pressure gauge). In contrast, tonometry involves the use of an external, noninvasive measurement to estimate IOP.

Tonometry has traditionally relied on a number of different strategies to estimate IOP. Schiøtz tonometers use indentation of the cornea with a weighted tip, and the degree of indentation is correlated with the IOP. Applanation tonometers, such as the Goldmann tonometer, use the Imbert-Fick principle, which models the cornea as a thin, flexible nondistensible sphere. When a flat applanation tip is placed against the surface of the eye, the pressure can be calculated based on the area applanated and the force required. The Mackay-Marg–type tonometers (eg, pneumatonometer, Tonopen) provide a point measurement of IOP based on the Mackay-Marg principle. With these devices, a tip with a moveable central piston is applanated against the cornea. As the tip is pressed against the eye, and the area of contact is progressively increased, this results in a characteristic pressure profile that increases, reaches a peak, dips to a trough, and then starts increasing again. The change in pressure from baseline to the trough provides the estimate of IOP.

Each of these types of tonometers has advantages and disadvantages, and several new types of devices attempt to address specific deficiencies.

Gedde SJ, ed. *Curbside Consultation in Glaucoma:*
49 Clinical Questions, Second Edition (pp 63–66)
© 2015 Taylor & Francis Group

Dynamic Contour Tonometry

One of the key limitations in the assessment of IOP has been the influence of central corneal thickness (CCT) and ocular rigidity. In general, the greater the deformation of the eye that is required, the greater the influence of ocular biomechanical properties on the IOP estimate. Dynamic contour tonometry (DCT) uses the principle that when an applanation tip is pressed against the surface of the eye, the pressure at the interface should be equal to the pressure inside the eye. However, if significant tissue deformation occurs, then ocular biomechanical properties start to affect measurements. To minimize this effect, DCT has a curved tip that approximately matches the cornea. When pressed against the eye, it results in "contour matching" that enables applanation with minimal tissue deformation. A pressure sensor at the middle of the applanation tip records the interface pressure continuously, enabling short tracing of the IOP to be measured. This approach appears to be effective in minimizing the effect of corneal thickness variations, allowing DCT to be particularly useful in patients with very thick or thin central corneas.[1]

Ocular Response Analyzer

The ocular response analyzer is a noncontact tonometer with software to analyze the additional parameters that may represent ocular biomechanical properties. When an air jet is used to indent the cornea, the rate at which it compresses is different from the rate at which it relaxes. This difference is described as the corneal hysteresis (CH) and is felt to be related to the viscoelastic damping of the eye. A second parameter, the corneal resistance factor (CRF), is also derived from the indentation vs pressure curve developed by the device and likely reflects overall ocular rigidity.[2] The value of these measures in clinical practice continues to be evaluated.

Two IOP measurements are produced by the device. The first is a pressure that is correlated to the expected Goldmann applanation tonometer (GAT) based on a normative database, and the second is a corneal compensated pressure that attempts to account for the individual corneal biomechanics. The corneal compensated pressure appears to be less affected by CCT than GAT.[3]

Rebound Tonometer

The rebound tonometer attempts to address the problem of requiring topical anesthetic for IOP measurements. Although noncontact tonometers do not require topical anesthetic, they can be difficult for patients who cannot position their head in the device or fixate adequately for the measurements. The rebound tonometer is a portable device that operates on the principle that an object projected at the corneal surface with a fixed velocity will decelerate and rebound faster if the IOP is higher.[4] The iCare tonometer (Icare Finland Oy, Vantaa, Finland) uses a small disposable probe with a permanent magnet that is propelled against the cornea using a solenoid, which also measures the probe deceleration. Since topical anesthetic is not required, and the device is portable, it may be particularly well suited for IOP measurements in younger children and infants and has potential utility in home IOP monitoring. The device is calibrated against GAT readings, and clinical studies suggest a reasonable correlation with GAT measurements.[5] However, since the technique depends on rebound from the cornea, it is significantly affected by corneal thickness with overestimates on eyes with thick corneas.[6]

Twenty-Four-Hour Measurement of Intraocular Pressure

Continuous 24-hour measurements of IOP can be categorized broadly into temporary and permanent approaches, two complementary but overlapping monitoring paradigms.[7] Temporary monitoring would necessarily involve noninvasive measurements of IOP, likely over a 24- to 48-hour period. Permanent monitoring would involve an implant that would enable IOP measurement over the life of the implant. Although continuous monitoring is technically feasible, current technology seems to favor periodic assessments limited to times when the devices can be powered externally and when the data can be read and stored.

Although both of these categories have a long history of research, only recently have devices for continuous monitoring of IOP started to appear in clinical use. Perhaps closest to common clinical use is the Triggerfish contact lens system (Sensimed AG, Lausanne, Switzerland), which is CE marked in Europe and can be used clinically, but is still undergoing clinical trials in the United States. This device uses a silicone contact lens with an embedded strain gauge to measure the change in corneal radius of curvature with IOP.[8] An embedded antenna allows the device to be powered wirelessly through induction and data to be transmitted to an external recorder. The contact lens is worn for a 24-hour period, allowing measurement of IOP patterns. The device appears to be well tolerated, and the IOP patterns are consistent with those from sleep laboratories.[9] However, the device is currently not calibrated to measure pressure in mm Hg, and the importance of evaluating IOP patterns alone remains to be demonstrated.

One of the main considerations with 24-hour measurement of IOP is how to integrate these data into clinical practice. The immediate role of 24-hour IOP monitoring will likely be to optimize the quality of IOP control in patients with glaucoma. A portion of patients with glaucoma continues to have disease progression despite seemingly well-controlled IOP when measured in the clinic. However, IOP variations, and not just mean IOP, may be a significant risk factor for glaucoma progression.[10–12] As well, sleep laboratory data have consistently shown that approximately two-thirds of patients have their highest IOP outside of office hours, with a peak typically occurring during sleep.[13] These patterns have been replicated with the Triggerfish contact lens system. Once a patient has been identified as having large IOP fluctuations or nocturnal elevation, appropriate therapy can be selected to flatten out IOP peaks across the 24-hour period. For example, prostaglandin analogues and carbonic anhydrase inhibitors appear to have better nocturnal efficacy than β-blockers or α-agonists. Treatments that improve outflow facility, such as laser trabeculoplasty and trabeculectomy, have an even greater effect on reducing IOP fluctuations. However, further work is required to fully understand the optimal IOP patterns for patients with glaucoma.

References

1. Kotecha A, White ET, Shewry JM, Garway-Heath DF. The relative effects of corneal thickness and age on Goldmann applanation tonometry and dynamic contour tonometry. *Br J Ophthalmol.* 2005;89(12):1572-1575.
2. Terai N, Raiskup F, Haustein M, et al. Identification of biomechanical properties of the cornea: the ocular response analyzer. *Curr Eye Res.* 2012;37(7):553-562.
3. Medeiros FA, Weinreb RN. Evaluation of the influence of corneal biomechanical properties on intraocular pressure measurements using the ocular response analyzer. *J Glaucoma.* 2006;15(5):364-370.
4. Kontiola AI. A new induction-based impact method for measuring intraocular pressure. *Acta Ophthalmol Scand.* 2000;78(2):142-145.
5. Cook JA, Botello AP, Elders A, et al. Systematic review of the agreement of tonometers with Goldmann applanation tonometry. *Ophthalmology.* 2012;119(8):1552-1557.

6. Nakamura M, Darhad U, Tatsumi Y, et al. Agreement of rebound tonometer in measuring intraocular pressure with three types of applanation tonometers. *Am J Ophthalmol.* 2006;142(2):332-334.

7. Sit AJ. Continuous monitoring of intraocular pressure: rationale and progress toward a clinical device. *J Glaucoma.* 2009;18(4):272-279.

8. Leonardi M, Leuenberger P, Bertrand D, et al. First steps toward noninvasive intraocular pressure monitoring with a sensing contact lens. *Invest Ophthalmol Vis Sci.* 2004;45(9):3113-3117.

9. Mansouri K, Medeiros FA, Tafreshi A, Weinreb RN. Continuous 24-hour monitoring of intraocular pressure patterns with a contact lens sensor: safety, tolerability, and reproducibility in patients with glaucoma. *Arch Ophthalmol.* 2012;130(12):1534-1539.

10. Caprioli J, Coleman AL. Intraocular pressure fluctuation a risk factor for visual field progression at low intraocular pressures in the advanced glaucoma intervention study. *Ophthalmology.* 2008;115(7):1123-1129.e3.

11. Musch DC, Gillespie BW, Niziol LM, et al. Intraocular pressure control and long-term visual field loss in the Collaborative Initial Glaucoma Treatment Study. *Ophthalmology.* 2011;118(9):1766-1773.

12. Asrani S, Zeimer R, Wilensky J, et al. Large diurnal fluctuations in intraocular pressure are an independent risk factor in patients with glaucoma. *J Glaucoma.* 2000;9(2):134-142.

13. Liu JH, Bouligny RP, Kripke DF, Weinreb RN. Nocturnal elevation of intraocular pressure is detectable in the sitting position. *Invest Ophthalmol Vis Sci.* 2003;44(10):4439-4442.

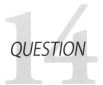

WHEN IS IMAGING OF THE ANTERIOR SEGMENT USEFUL?

Michael Banitt, MD and
Anne Ko, MD

Imaging of the anterior segment can be used to confirm diagnoses for which clinical suspicion already exists. This chapter discusses the anterior segment imaging modalities that are most relevant to the care of the patient with glaucoma.

Ultrasound biomicroscopy (UBM) produces higher resolution images than does standard ultrasound. It can be used to image virtually all anterior segment structures (and visually apparent pathology), including the cornea (Descemet's membrane detachments), anterior chamber angle (narrow angles), iris (cysts, iridodialysis, and melanomas), ciliary body (cyclodialysis clefts and melanomas), and lens (residual lens fragments, poorly positioned intraocular lens [IOL] haptics and optics, and abnormal lens shapes). UBM is the imaging modality that best provides images of structures that lie within and deep to pigmented tissues.

UBM has long been used to objectively evaluate the anterior chamber angle (ACA) and is highly correlated with gonioscopic findings in this respect.[1-3] It can be used to confirm narrow angles, angle closure, and deepening of the angle after an iridotomy. In patients with hypotony, it can be used to verify the existence of a cyclodialysis cleft or cyclitic membrane. Unlike gonioscopy, UBM cannot be used to determine whether subtle ACA characteristics such as anterior synechiae and/or neovascularization exist. UBM is, however, an effective imaging modality for those patients who have cloudy corneas or who are intolerant to gonioscopy.

There are several clinical scenarios in which UBM can clarify gonioscopic findings. Specifically, UBM should be performed in cases where angles are asymmetric, in patients with focal peripheral anterior synechiae in the setting of an otherwise open angle, and also in eyes suspected to have anteriorly rotated ciliary bodies. In these situations, UBM can aid in the diagnosis of iris cysts or masses and plateau iris. Because it can image structures within and deep to pigmented tissues, UBM is the best modality with which to capture iris cysts that generally appear as thin, rounded reflective walls with sonolucent, fluid-filled interiors. In contrast, iris and ciliary body melanomas

Gedde SJ, ed. *Curbside Consultation in Glaucoma:*
49 Clinical Questions, Second Edition (pp 67–69)
© 2015 Taylor & Francis Group

typically exhibit homogeneous patterns of low to moderate reflectivity. Importantly, UBM can also be used to determine whether an iris melanoma has extended into the ciliary body.

In the setting of persistent unexplained inflammation after cataract surgery, UBM can be used to detect retained nuclear fragments located deep to the iris plane. In cases where uveitis glaucoma hyphema syndrome (UGH) is suspected or in patients with persistent postoperative pain, UBM can determine whether a poorly positioned IOL is the cause.

To obtain a reasonable balance between image resolution and depth of tissue penetration, the most widely used commercial UBM models rely on 50-MHz transducers. Since these transducers require the use of a coupling medium, UBMs can be time consuming and inconvenient to perform. As a result, noncontact imagining modalities have been developed. The alternatives include optical coherence tomography (OCT) and Scheimpflug photography.

OCT is a high-resolution, optically based imaging system that uses low-coherence interferometry to provide cross-sectional images of ocular tissue. Both OCT and UBM have advantages over gonioscopy in that they can be performed under truly dark conditions, and they lack the interobserver variability that characterizes gonioscopy. A modification to the standard posterior segment OCT, the use of a 1310-nm infrared light source, allows for improved penetration through nontransparent anterior segment structures. So, although UBM is preferred, anterior segment (AS)–OCT can be used to evaluate iris cysts and small hypopigmented iris tumors that are located anterior to the pigmented epithelium.[4] It cannot evaluate structures located behind the pigmented epithelium.

Evidence suggests that the AS-OCT can be used to objectively assess and document the depth of the ACA.[5,6] In this regard, its findings have been highly correlated to gonioscopy and UBM, both of which require prolonged patient cooperation and contact with the eye (as well as fluid coupling in the case of UBM). Like UBM but unlike gonioscopy, AS-OCT cannot capture the presence of peripheral anterior synechiae and/or neovascularization. However, in eyes with type 1 Boston keratoprostheses, the AS-OCT has been shown to be more effective than UBM in following progressive ACA closure.

In the past, AS-OCT has been used to statically evaluate the anterior chamber. However, the Fourier domain AS-OCT now allows for the capture of large volumes of data by rapidly and 3-dimensionally cube scanning the anterior segment. By evaluating all 360 degrees of the anterior chamber, it is possible to determine the volume of the iris and anterior chamber. In the future, being able to quantify changes in iris area and volume may allow for better identification of eyes that are at risk for acute angle closure.

Finally, specular and confocal microscopy can play a role in the evaluation of a very small subset of patients with glaucoma. Patients with iridocorneal endothelial syndrome will pathognomonically exhibit a unilateral "dark light reversal" in which their epithelial-like endothelial cells appear to have bright boundaries, dark cell bodies, and nuclei that give off a bright signal. Unaffected endothelial cells exhibit dark cell boundaries with bright cell bodies and unrecognizable nuclei.

Summary

Gonioscopy remains the gold standard for examining visible parts of the anterior segment. While UBM and AS-OCT have several advantages over gonioscopy, they typically play an adjunct role in the management of patients with glaucoma except in cases where gonioscopy is not possible or structures are not visible. UBM and OCT can also be used in patient education and to illustrate treatment success (although this alone does not justify additional testing).

References

1. Friedman DS, Gazzard G, Foster P, et al. Ultrasonographic biomicroscopy, Scheimpflug photography, and novel provocative tests in contralateral eyes of Chinese patients initially seen with acute angle closure. *Arch Ophthalmol.* 2003;121(5):633-642.
2. Friedman DS, Gazzard G, Min CB, et al. Age and sex variation in angle findings among normal Chinese subjects: a comparison of UBM, Scheimpflug, and gonioscopic assessment of the anterior chamber angle. *J Glaucoma.* 2008;17(1):5-10.
3. Kurita N, Mayama C, Tomidokoro A, Aihara M, Araie M. Potential of the pentacam in screening for primary angle closure and primary angle closure suspect. *J Glaucoma.* 2009;18(7):506-512.
4. Pavlin CJ, Vasquez LM, Lee R, Simpson ER, Ahmed II. Anterior segment optical coherence tomography and ultrasound biomicroscopy in the imaging of anterior segment tumors. *Am J Ophthalmol.* 2009;147(2):214-219.e2.
5. Pekmezci M, Porco TC, Lin SC. Anterior segment optical coherence tomography as a screening tool for the assessment of the anterior segment angle. *Ophthalmic Surg Lasers Imaging.* 2009;40(4):389-398.
6. Radhakrishnan S, Goldsmith J, Huang D, et al. Comparison of optical coherence tomography and ultrasound biomicroscopy for detection of narrow anterior chamber angles. *Arch Ophthalmol.* 2005;123(8):1053-1059.

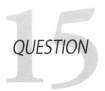

IN WHICH PATIENTS WITH GLAUCOMA SHOULD I PERFORM NEUROIMAGING, CARDIOVASCULAR EVALUATION, AND/OR LABORATORY TESTING?

David S. Greenfield, MD

Various nonglaucomatous disorders may produce optic disc cupping and visual field disturbances that resemble the clinical profile of normal-tension glaucoma (NTG), and it is important
that clinicians recognize them. These disorders (Figure 15-1) include hereditary optic neuropathy,
antecedent optic nerve infarction, trauma, syphilis, demyelinating optic neuritis, fusiform enlargement of the intracranial carotid artery, and intraorbital and intracranial mass lesions. Although
Trobe and colleagues[1] reported that pallor of the neuroretinal rim was 94% specific in predicting
nonglaucomatous cupping, and focal or diffuse obliteration of the neuroretinal rim was 87% specific in predicting glaucomatous cupping, clinically differentiating these disorders from glaucoma
remains a subjective and often difficult challenge. Thus, ancillary tests have been proposed in the
diagnostic evaluation of NTG (Table 15-1).

Neuroimaging

Anecdotal reports have described occult intracranial mass lesions simulating glaucomatous
nerve fiber bundle visual field defects, and neuroimaging has been suggested by some authors to
exclude such lesions. Greenfield and colleagues[2] evaluated the incidence of positive neuroradiologic studies among consecutive patients with NTG who underwent cranial neuroimaging as part
of a diagnostic evaluation over a 10-year period. None of the patients diagnosed with glaucoma
had neuroradiologic evidence of a mass lesion involving the anterior visual pathway. A masked
analysis of optic disc photographs and visual fields was performed among patients with NTG and
a control group of eyes with optic disc cupping associated with compressive visual pathway lesions.
Age younger than 50 years, visual acuity below 20/40, vertically aligned visual field defects, and

Gedde SJ, ed. *Curbside Consultation in Glaucoma:*
49 Clinical Questions, Second Edition (pp 71–75)
© 2015 Taylor & Francis Group

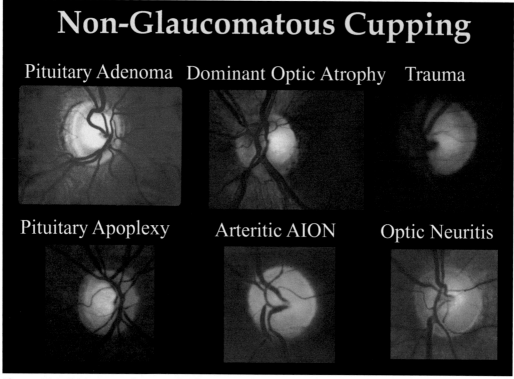

Figure 15-1. Optic nerve photographs illustrate various mechanisms of nonglaucomatous disorders that may produce optic disc cupping and visual field disturbances that resemble the clinical profile of glaucomatous optic neuropathy.

pallor of the neural rim were found to be highly specific for nonglaucomatous cupping. Patients with these clinical features should undergo neuroimaging.

Cardiovascular Evaluation

Vascular risk factors have been well described in NTG and include migraine headache and disc hemorrhage, peripheral vasospasm, systemic hypotension or previous hemodynamic crisis, nocturnal dips in blood pressure, reduced orbital blood flow velocity, and cranial magnetic resonance imaging abnormalities suggestive of ischemia. Some investigators have found significantly increased ipsilateral carotid artery resistive indices in eyes with asymmetric glaucomatous visual field loss. These observations have led many to pursue ancillary diagnostic tests in the evaluation of NTG such as carotid Doppler and laboratory examination to exclude the possibility of comorbid conditions such as carotid stenosis, arteritis, hyperviscosity syndromes, and anemia.

Limited information exists regarding the prevalence of carotid Doppler abnormalities among persons with glaucoma. O'Brien et al[3] evaluated 12 eyes with asymmetric primary open-angle glaucoma (POAG) and found significantly increased ipsilateral carotid artery resistive indices in eyes with advanced glaucomatous visual field loss. In contrast, Jampol and Miller[4] evaluated 5 eyes with severe carotid stenosis and ocular hypertension. No glaucomatous disc damage was observed at 3 to 12 years of longitudinal follow-up. Greenfield and Bagga[5] evaluated the prevalence of hemodynamically significant (>70%) carotid artery stenosis in a pilot study among 20 persons with

Table 15-1
Ancillary Tests in the
Diagnostic Evaluation of Normal Tension Glaucoma

Test	Symptoms	Ocular Signs
Brain/orbital MRI	Unexplained visual loss	Optic disc pallor or edema, 20/40 acuity or worse, vertically aligned visual field defect, proptosis
Carotid Doppler	Transient visual obscuration (amaurosis fugax)	Retinal emboli, iris or retinal neovascularization, midperipheral intraretinal hemorrhage
ESR, C-reactive protein	Temporal headache, jaw claudication, scalp tenderness, weight loss, muscle pain	Optic disc pallor or edema, retinal artery occlusion, reduced temporal artery pulse with tenderness or induration
CBC	History of anemia or recent blood loss	Optic disc pallor, retinal hemorrhage
VDRL, FTA-ABS	History of syphilis, reduced vision	Optic disc pallor or edema, uveitis or chorioretinitis, vasculitis, interstitial keratitis

Abbreviations: CBC, complete blood count; ESR, erythrocyte sedimentation rate ; FTA-ABS, fluorescent treponemal antibody absorption; MRI, magnetic resonance imaging; VDRL, veneral disease research laboratory.

glaucoma. Patients were subdivided into 2 groups based on glaucoma subtype (normal-tension vs primary open-angle glaucoma [POAG]) and severity (mild = visual field mean deviation [MD] ≤ 6 dB vs moderate-advanced = MD > 6 dB). The magnitude of carotid stenosis (Figure 15-2) was similar in eyes with NTG and POAG, and the severity of glaucomatous damage as determined by visual field MD did not correlate with the degree of carotid artery stenosis. Glaucomatous cupping and visual field loss as an isolated manifestation of carotid stenosis is uncommon, and I recommend a targeted approach in selected patients with transient visual obscuration, retinal emboli, or signs of ocular ischemia.

Laboratory Evaluation

Studies[6] have suggested a greater prevalence of immune-related phenomenon among patients with NTG. Wax and colleagues[7] identified a greater prevalence of serum monoclonal proteins and autoantibodies to extractable nuclear antigens (such as Sjögren syndrome A antigen) among 44 patients with NTG compared with 41 patients with POAG. In contrast, other studies[5] have reported no differences in serum laboratory testing (erythrocyte sedimentation rate, complete

Figure 15-2. Distribution of carotid stenosis grade (mild = 0% to 39%, moderate = 40% to 69%, severe = 70% to 100%) demonstrates a similar prevalence (*P* = .8) among patients with NTG and POAG. (Reprinted with permission from Greenfield DS, Bagga H. Blood flow studies and serological testing in the diagnostic evaluation of glaucoma: a pilot study. *Ophthalmic Surg Lasers Imaging.* 2004;35:406-414.)

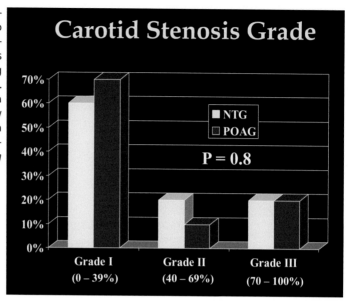

blood count, veneral disease research laboratory [VDRL], and fluorescent treponemal antibody absorption [FTA-ABS]) between patients with NTG and POAG. I do not perform routine serum laboratory testing in all patients with NTG.

Summary

Younger age, reduced central vision, abnormal color vision, optic disc pallor disproportionate to the degree of cupping, and vertically aligned visual field defects represent risk factors for compression intracranial lesions and are indications for neuroimaging. There is insufficient evidence to suggest that patients with NTG should undergo routine neurodiagnostic, vascular, or serum laboratory examination. A comprehensive history and ocular examination will assist the clinician in targeting persons in whom such testing is warranted.

Acknowledgment

Supported in part by the Maltz Family Endowment for Glaucoma Research, Cleveland, Ohio, and a grant from Barney Donnelley, Palm Beach, Florida.

References

1. Trobe JD, Glaser JS, Cassady J, Herschler J, Anderson DR. Nonglaucomatous excavation of the optic disc. *Arch Ophthalmol.* 1980;98:1046-1050.
2. Greenfield DS, Siatkowski RM, Glaser JS, Schatz NJ, Parrish RK. The cupped disc: who needs neuroimaging? *Ophthalmology.* 1998;105:1866-1874.
3. O'Brien C, Saxton V, Crick RP, Meire H. Doppler carotid artery studies in asymmetric glaucoma. *Eye.* 1992;6:273.
4. Jampol LM, Miller NR. Carotid artery disease and glaucoma. *Br J Ophthalmol.* 1978;62:324.

5. Greenfield DS, Bagga H. Blood flow studies and serological testing in the diagnostic evaluation of glaucoma: a pilot study. *Ophthalmic Surg Lasers Imaging.* 2004;35:406-414.

6. Cartwright M, Grajewski AL, Friedberg ML, Anderson DR, Richards DW. Immune-related disease and normal-tension glaucoma, a case control study. *Arch Ophthalmol.* 1992;110:500-502.

7. Wax MB, Barrett DA, Pestronk A. Increased incidence of paraproteinemia and autoantibodies in patients with normal-tension glaucoma. *Am J Ophthalmol.* 1994;117:561-568.

IS GENETIC TESTING USEFUL IN SCREENING IN GLAUCOMA?

John H. Fingert, MD, PhD

Heredity has an important role in the pathogenesis of primary open-angle glaucoma (POAG). Many studies of twins, families, populations, and inbred animals have shown that POAG has a strong genetic basis. More recently, scientists have identified some of the specific genes that cause POAG. Consequently, there has been great interest in using genetic testing to aid with early detection of POAG and early institution of currently available treatments.

Some cases of POAG are caused in part by the combined action of many genetic risk factors. These glaucoma risk factors are observed at a significantly higher frequency in patients with POAG than in normal individuals. However, each risk factor contributes very small risk for the development of glaucoma and cannot cause disease on its own. For example, a genetic variation near the caveolin 1 and caveolin 2 genes (*rs4236601*) has been detected in 28.8% of a large cohort of patients with POAG and 22.8% of matched controls from Iceland ($P = 5.0 \times 10^{-10}$). These data suggest that variants in the caveolin 1 or caveolin 2 gene may be associated with increased risk for POAG (odds ratio, 1.36) but are unable to cause glaucoma on their own.[1] Due to the large number of independently inherited factors that must work in concert to promote disease, this form of POAG does not have a discernable inheritance pattern but instead may be seen to cluster within families or ethnic populations. Currently, more than a dozen glaucoma genetic risk factors have been discovered, including *CAV1/2*, *CDKN2B-AS1*, *TMCO1*, *SIX1/6*, *ATOH7*, *SRBD1*, *ELOVL5*, and *TLR4*. The role of genetic testing for these risk factors has recently been addressed by the American Academy of Ophthalmology (AAO) with guidelines for the use of genetic testing in eye disease. The Academy recommends that routine genetic testing for late-onset POAG be avoided until strong evidence is provided that testing will help guide the selection of glaucoma therapies.[2] Each of the aforementioned genetic factors contributes too little risk for POAG for testing to be useful or predictive. However, testing may be warranted in the future when more genetic risk

Gedde SJ, ed. *Curbside Consultation in Glaucoma:*
49 Clinical Questions, Second Edition (pp 77–79)
© 2015 Taylor & Francis Group

factors for glaucoma have been discovered, which may allow tests for multiple factors in combination to have more predictive value for likely prognosis or response to available therapies.

Other cases of POAG have simple, autosomal dominant inheritance patterns and appear to be caused primarily by a single gene. Patients with this type of POAG are often part of large pedigrees with many family members who have glaucoma. Genetic studies have provided strong evidence that mutations in 3 genes—myocilin, optineurin, and *TBK1*—may cause POAG. Mutations in myocilin are associated with 3% to 4% of POAG that frequently presents with elevated intraocular pressure (IOP). Mutations in either optineurin or *TBK1* are associated with 1% to 3% of POAG that occurs at low IOP. Individuals who inherit a mutation in one of these glaucoma genes almost always develop glaucoma, and consequently, glaucoma-causing mutations in these genes are almost never seen in normal individuals. Other POAG genes have been reported (*WDR36*, *NTF4*, and *ASB10*), but the role of these genes in glaucoma pathogenesis is controversial.[3]

Genetic testing for myocilin is widely available and can be arranged via many laboratories (www.genetests.org). However, given the low prevalence of myocilin, optineurin, and *TBK1* mutations in unselected patients with POAG (< 4%), testing of unselected cases of glaucoma is not advisable due to the low rate of positive tests. However, select patient groups are more likely to have mutations in these genes as described below. When identified, genetic testing for these high-risk groups may be helpful as part of a surveillance plan as well as for selecting a treatment regimen.

- Myoclin genetic testing: Patients with POAG who are diagnosed at a young age (ie, < 40 years of age), have a markedly elevated IOP (ie, > 30 mm Hg), and have a strong family history of glaucoma may benefit from genetic testing for a myocilin mutation. Detection of specific myocilin mutations may help physicians select the best therapies for their patients. Some myocilin mutations (ie, *TYR437HIS*) are associated with a rapidly progressive form of glaucoma that responds poorly to medical management. Early surgical intervention in such patients may be indicated (Figure 16-1). POAG caused by other myocilin mutations (ie, *GLN368STOP*) often responds well to medical therapies and may not require early surgical interventions.[4] Individuals with relatives who have glaucoma due to previously detected myocilin mutations are at high risk for carrying the same myocilin mutations and might also benefit from testing. In such individuals, a positive test result would help focus screening examinations on those at highest risk as well as help with the selection of treatment options. A negative test would allow reassurance that an individual does not carry the family's higher risk for POAG and might allow screening efforts to be focused on people at higher risk for developing glaucoma.

- Optineurin genetic testing: Genetic testing for optineurin mutations is also not advisable for unselected patients with POAG. Those patients who are most likely to have an optineurin mutation have a strong family history of normal-tension glaucoma (NTG) and an early age at diagnosis. Similarly, members of a family with a known glaucoma-causing optineurin mutation might benefit from testing.

- TBK1 genetic testing: *TBK1* genetic testing is not currently available for clinical use.

Finally, it is vital that genetic testing be ordered by experienced physicians and/or genetic counselors who have the capabilities to properly interpret test results and explain them to their patients.

References

1. Thorleifsson G, Walters GB, Hewitt AW, et al. Common variants near CAV1 and CAV2 are associated with primary open-angle glaucoma. *Nat Genet*. 2010;42(10):906-909.

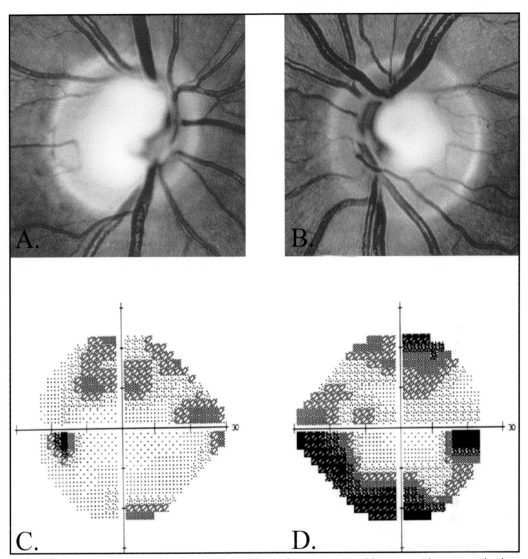

Figure 16-1. Disc photos and Humphrey visual field tests from a 27-year-old patient with open-angle glaucoma (OAG) associated with a *TYR437HIS* mutation in myocilin. This patient has typical features of myocilin-associated glaucoma, including an early age at diagnosis of glaucoma (25 years), a strong family history of glaucoma (> 20 family members with glaucoma), and a high maximum IOP (40 mm Hg OD and 30 mm Hg OS). She has asymmetric cupping OD > OS. There is superior thinning of the neural rim OD (A) and a corresponding inferior arcuate visual field defect (D). Cupping OS is less prominent (B) and associated with an early superior arcuate defect (C).

2. Stone EM, Aldave AJ, Drack AV, et al. Recommendations for genetic testing of inherited eye diseases: report of the American Academy of Ophthalmology task force on genetic testing. *Ophthalmology.* 2012;119(11):2408-2410.

3. Fingert JH. Primary open-angle glaucoma genes. *Eye.* 2011;25(5):587-595.

4. Graul TA, Kwon YH, Zimmerman MB, et al. A case-control comparison of the clinical characteristics of glaucoma and ocular hypertensive patients with and without the myocilin Gln368Stop mutation. *Am J Ophthalmol.* 2002;134(6):884-890.

HOW IS CEREBROSPINAL FLUID PRESSURE RELATED TO GLAUCOMA?

David Fleischman, MD, MS and
R. Rand Allingham, MD

Primary open-angle glaucoma (POAG) is one of the most common forms of glaucoma worldwide. A growing body of evidence implicates cerebrospinal fluid pressure (CSFP) as an important factor in the pathogenesis of glaucoma. Let us briefly review what we know about this illness. Glaucoma is typified by characteristic optic nerve damage and corresponding visual field loss. Intraocular pressure (IOP) is arguably the most important risk factor for glaucoma; not surprisingly, the only current therapies for glaucoma are interventions that reduce IOP. The normal-tension form of primary open-angle glaucoma (NTG) and ocular hypertension (OHT) complicates our understanding of the role of IOP in this disease. In patients with NTG, nerve damage and field loss occur despite historically recorded IOP in the "normal" range. It has also been shown that reduction of IOP below the patient's baseline IOP delays or prevents progression. The case of OHT is similarly interesting, if not confusing. The Ocular Hypertensive Treatment Study (OHTS) found that approximately 9% of patients with OHT would eventually develop glaucomatous change in the optic nerve, visual field, or both within 5 years.[1] This means that most patients with an IOP above "normal" may never go on to develop glaucomatous disease. These data underscore the notion that in addition to IOP, there remain important undiscovered risk factors for glaucoma.

There is a growing interest in the role of CSFP in POAG. One reason for this is the anatomy of the lamina cribrosa and surrounding tissues. The lamina cribrosa is the thin piece of scleral tissue where the axons of the retinal ganglion cells exit the eye. This tissue serves as the boundary between 2 differentially pressurized compartments—the intraocular space containing the aqueous humor and the subarachnoid space containing the cerebrospinal fluid (CSF). This is the site of retinal ganglion cell injury by mechanical obstruction of axonal axoplasmic flow, vascular insufficiency, or other causes. A number of studies have investigated the retrolaminar tissue pressure in the pathogenesis of glaucoma with mixed results.[2-4] More recent studies, by Morgan et al,[5] have

Gedde SJ, ed. *Curbside Consultation in Glaucoma:*
49 Clinical Questions, Second Edition (pp 81–84)
© 2015 Taylor & Francis Group

Figure 17-1. The presumed relationship between CSFP and glaucoma and increased IOP. The lamina cribrosa serves as the boundary between the 2 differentially pressurized compartments. (Reprinted with permission from Fleischman D, Allingham RR. The role of CSFP in glaucoma and other ophthalmic diseases: a review. *Saudi J Ophthal.* 2013;27:97-106.)

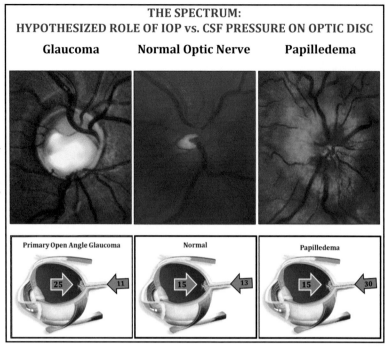

THE SPECTRUM:
HYPOTHESIZED ROLE OF IOP vs. CSF PRESSURE ON OPTIC DISC
Glaucoma   Normal Optic Nerve   Papilledema

Primary Open Angle Glaucoma   Normal   Papilledema

performed biomechanical studies to examine the response of the lamina cribrosa to changes in IOP and CSFP in the dog model. These studies in the pressure difference across the lamina cribrosa (the translaminar pressure difference) have supported the concept that changes in CSFP induce tissue movement (strain) in this tissue that may be important in the pathology of glaucoma. Specifically, elevated IOP and decreased CSFP produce force that causes posterior bowing of the lamina cribrosa seen in glaucoma. The reverse is also true: anteriorly directed force caused by increased CSFP causes anterior bowing of the lamina cribrosa, consistent with what is observed in patients with papilledema (Figure 17-1).

Berdahl and colleagues[6] studied this theory clinically for the first time. Patients with POAG had lower CSFP than did control patients. Patients with normal-tension glaucoma had even lower pressures than did patients with POAG, and interestingly, patients with OHT had higher CSFP than did the control patients. Ren et al[7] studied this in prospective fashion and observed strikingly similar results. The implication is that a low CSFP, by increasing the translaminar pressure difference, may increase forces across the lamina cribrosa that contribute to glaucomatous injury. Conversely, ocular hypertensives who have elevated CSFP may be protected against glaucoma by reducing the translaminar pressure difference.

If CSFP is not only a risk factor but also a pathogenic mechanism for glaucoma, could it possibly explain other well-known glaucoma risk factors? Age is another major risk factor for glaucoma in all populations studied to date. We examined the effect of age on CSFP in a large-scale retrospective study of more than 14, 000 individuals with a history of lumbar puncture and no known cause of elevated CSFP and a normal CSF fluid analysis. We found that the average CSFP is stable for the first 5 decades of life, after which there is a steady decline that extends through the 10th decade of life (Figure 17-2). The age at which CSF pressure begins to decrease coincides with the increase in prevalence of POAG. This finding offers a possible explanation for increased risk of POAG with age.

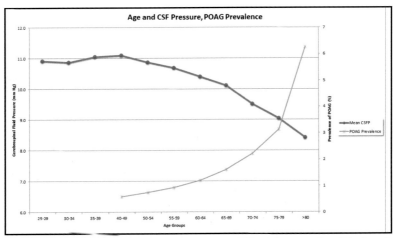

Figure 17-2. The relationship between average CFP and age against Friedman's meta-analysis of POAG prevalence (Friedman DS, Wolfs RC, O'Colmain BJ, et al. Prevalence of open-angle glaucoma (OAG) among adults in the United States. *Archives of Ophthalmology*. 2004 Apr;122(4):532-8.) Reprinted with permission from Fleischman D, Allingham RR. The role of CFP in glaucoma and other ophthalmic diseases: a review. *Saudi J Ophthal*. 2013;27:97-106.

Systemic blood pressure, particularly lower blood pressure, is a well-known risk factor for POAG. The role of reduced ocular perfusion pressure has been investigated in the past as well. Interestingly, blood pressure has been shown to positively correlate closely with CSFP. Therefore, it is possible that lower blood pressure, as well as its effect on ocular perfusion pressure, may exert an increased risk for POAG through its association with lower CSFP.

Body mass index (BMI) is another factor related to POAG risk. Low BMI has been suggested as a risk for the development of POAG, while increased BMI may be protective. Interestingly, CSFP is positively associated with BMI. If elevated CSFP is protective for POAG, then higher BMI would be consistent with this observation.

The data relating to the effect of CSFP on glaucoma risk are intriguing. However, the obvious question is, how can we measure this in our patients? Clearly, the data at this point do not support the use of lumbar puncture (LP) measurements for CSFP in the management of glaucoma. However, in the future, we may be able to use noninvasive approaches to infer CSFP. If clinicians are able to approximate a patient's CSFP status, this value could be used to calculate POAG risk, much like central corneal thickness (CCT) is used today. Currently, studies are being used to approximate CSF pressure by magnetic resonance neuroimaging of the optic nerve sheath. Other studies are investigating the use of ultrasound, or ultrasound biomicroscopy (UBM) or noninvasive technologies to study CSFP-related behavior of retinal blood vessels.

Other interesting issues pertain to CSF dynamics, such as the effect of positional changes on CSFP. For example, CSFP is routinely measured in the supine position. This is a static measure of a dynamically pressurized compartment. CSFP measured by a lumbar tap accurately represents intracranial pressure in the lateral decubitus position. However, in the upright position, intracranial pressure falls, possibly to subzero values. Furthermore, CSF dynamics with the orbital compartment are thought to differ from the rest of the neuraxis. Nevertheless, this compartment is continuous with the rest of the neural axis, as optic nerve sheath diameter has been found to increase with lumbar CSF infusion and after blood patching for CSF leaks. When calculating the translaminar pressure difference, investigators currently use supine CSF opening pressures with sitting position IOP measurements. Actual translaminar pressure differences are a dynamic process that includes instantaneous IOP, optic sheath pressure, and orbital pressures. Future studies will need to take these variables into account to apply these data clinically. While not yet clinically useful, understanding the role of intracranial pressure as it pertains to the pathogenesis of glaucoma may help stratify our patients' risk factors and affect our expectations with regard to response of treatment.

References

1. Kass MA, Heuer DK, Higginbotham EJ, Johnson CA, Keltner JL, Miller JP, Parrish RK, Wilson MR, Gordon MO. The Ocular Hypertension Treatment Study: a randomized trial determines that topical ocular hypotensive medication delays or prevents the onset of primary open-angle glaucoma. *Arch Ophthalmol.* 2002 Jun;120(6):701-713.
2. Yang Y, Yu M, Zhu J, Chen X, Liu X. Role of cerebrospinal fluid in glaucoma: pressure and beyond. Medical hypotheses. 2010 Jan;74(1):31-34.
3. Morgan WH, Chauhan BC, Yu DY, Cringle SJ, Alder VA, House PH. Optic disc movement with variations in intraocular and cerebrospinal fluid pressure. *Invest Ophthalmol Vis Sci.* 2002 Oct;43(10):3236-3242.
4. Morgan WH, Yu DY, Alder VA, Cringle SJ, Cooper RL, House PH, et al. The correlation between cerebrospinal fluid pressure and retrolaminar tissue pressure. *Invest Ophthalmol Vis Sci.* 1998 Jul;39(8):1419-1428.
5. Morgan WH, Yu DY, Cooper RL, Alder VA, Cringle SJ, Constable IJ. The influence of cerebrospinal fluid pressure on the lamina cribrosa tissue pressure gradient. *Invest Ophthalmol Vis Sci.* 1995 May;36(6):1163-1172.
6. Berdahl JP, Fautsch MP, Stinnett SS, Allingham RR. Intracranial pressure in primary open angle glaucoma, normal tension glaucoma, and ocular hypertension: a case-control study. *Invest Ophthalmol Vis Sci.* 2008;49(12):5412-5418.
7. Ren R, Jonas JB, Tian G, et al. Cerebrospinal fluid pressure in glaucoma: a prospective study. *Ophthalmology.* 2010;117(2):259-266.

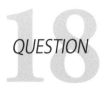

Do Anti-Vascular Endothelial Growth Factor Injections Cause Intraocular Pressure Elevation?

John T. Lind, MD, MS and
Andrew J. Barkmeier, MD

Since the introduction of intravitreal anti-vascular endothelial growth factor (anti-VEGF) therapy in 2005 with off-label bevacizumab and the subsequent Food and Drug Administration (FDA) approval of ranibizumab in 2006, the number of intravitreal injections has increased rapidly from several thousand annually to over 1 million injections every year in the United States. Initially approved for neovascular age-related macular degeneration (AMD), indications for intravitreal anti-VEGF therapy have since expanded to include diabetic macular edema, proliferative diabetic retinopathy, macular edema due to retinal vein occlusion, neovascular glaucoma, and others.

Sustained intraocular pressure (IOP) elevation has been reported following serial intravitreal injections, and two general pathogenic mechanisms have been proposed for this development. The first possibility relates to the transient but often dramatic postinjection pressure increase that results from the eye wall's limited elastic capability to respond to the increased intraocular volume. Ocular outflow structures may be damaged by either mechanical stretching or by the pressure rise itself. Alternatively, the trabecular meshwork or other outflow structures may be damaged, inflamed, or occluded by the injected medication itself, by other compounds in the vehicle, or by protein aggregates or contaminants such as silicone oil from the syringe. These potential mechanisms are still under active investigation.

Gedde SJ, ed. *Curbside Consultation in Glaucoma:*
49 Clinical Questions, Second Edition (pp 85–88)
© 2015 Taylor & Francis Group

Is There an Acute Intraocular Pressure Rise After Injection?

Yes. An immediate postinjection mean IOP elevation to 44 mm Hg was reported in a large series of consecutive injections by Kim et al,[1] with a range of 4 to 87 mm Hg. One patient developed acute transient vision loss to less than hand motions vision related to pressure-induced hypoperfusion. Risk factors for significant initial pressure elevation in this report were smaller needle bore size and preexisting glaucoma. Within 15 minutes of injection, 96% of eyes had an IOP less than 30 mm Hg, and all eyes were below this level within 30 minutes. Patients with glaucoma had a slower time to normalization of their IOP.

In the pivotal MARINA trail, Rosenfeld et al[2] found mean one hour postinjection IOP elevations of 1.9 to 3.5 and 2.1 to 3.4 mm Hg in the two treatment (injection) groups compared with a change of 0.8 to 1.5 mm Hg in the sham injection group. Interestingly, pressures of 30 mm Hg or more were measured in 13.0% and 17.6% of the injection groups compared with only 3.4% of eyes after sham injection. There were no eyes with IOP measurements over 40 mm Hg after sham injection. However, pressures of 40 mm Hg or more and 50 mm Hg or more were found in 2.3% and 0.6% of eyes, respectively, following intravitreal anti-VEGF injections. Patients with glaucoma were not excluded from this trial unless pressures were greater than 30 mm Hg despite pressure-lowering treatment.

Is There Risk of Prolonged Pressure Elevation Following Serial Anti-VEGF Injections?

Choi et al[3] reported an approximate 10% incidence of sustained IOP elevation over 25 mm Hg in their large series of patients without underlying glaucoma who had received serial anti-VEGF injections. There was no correlation found between the number or frequency of injections and the likelihood of IOP elevation in their patient population.

Hoang et al[4] similarly found that 11.6% of patients without preexisting ocular hypertension or glaucoma developed sustained IOP elevation (defined as an increase >5 mm Hg) following serial injections. In this study, however, a larger number of injections were associated with an increased risk of pressure elevation.

What Are Our Recommendations for Monitoring for Intraocular Pressure Elevations Following Anti-VEGF Treatment?

When anti-VEGF treatment is considered, it is important to assess the patient's optic disc and evaluate his or her ability to tolerate wide fluctuations in IOPs. For patients without underlying glaucoma, the optic nerve will typically tolerate temporary, modest pressure elevations. Patients with advanced glaucoma and visual field deficits approaching fixation, however, may be at significantly elevated risk for disease progression and could potentially "snuff out" their remaining central vision after beginning injections. It is important to review and document past glaucoma surgical history for anti-VEGF treatment candidates, as patients with preexisting tube shunt or

Table 18-1
Important Factors to Consider in Patients Receiving Intravitreal Injections
Six questions I ask myself when encountering a patient who needs repeat anti-VEGF injections:
1. Does this patient have underlying glaucoma?
2. Has there been progression of the visual field or progressive cupping of the nerve?
3. Is there a trend in progressive elevation of his or her intraocular pressure?
4. Has the patient undergone an ab externo filtering procedure (trabeculectomy or tube shunt)?
5. Should I be following this patient more closely?
6. Am I communicating with the patient's retina specialist?

trabeculectomy procedures may have some protection from volume expansion and outflow inhibition.

It is the combined responsibility of the retina specialist, glaucoma specialist, and comprehensive ophthalmologist to discuss the risks of ocular hypertension and glaucomatous progression with the patient while he or she is receiving intravitreal anti-VEGF injections. It is critical to stress the importance of continuing close glaucoma follow-up despite the increased frequency of their visits to the retina specialist. We recommend that patients with underlying glaucoma who are receiving serial anti-VEGF injections be followed more closely than the established Preferred Practice Pattern recommendation of every 3 to 6 months. Assessing the optic nerve head status at every glaucoma appointment and checking visual fields more regularly in these patients is paramount. The severity of the underlying glaucoma, above goal IOPs, and progression of visual field defects or progressive optic nerve head cupping would be indications for advancement of treatment and even closer monitoring.

Communication between the retina specialist and glaucoma specialist is critical. Some patients may require alteration of a retina specialist's standard injection location to avoid needle penetration through areas of low, diffuse filtration blebs. Other patients at particularly high risk for glaucomatous progression may benefit from either low-volume injections (< 0.05 cc) or anterior chamber paracentesis to avoid extreme pressure elevations.

From a glaucoma specialist's standpoint, I like to ask patients themselves to take note of their pre- and postinjection IOPs. This can better help me assess the patient's risk for both injection-related and sustained pressure elevation-related damage. If I fear these pressures are higher than the eye can tolerate or there are signs of progressive damage such as enlarged cupping or confirmed visual field changes, advancing medical or surgical treatment may be recommended (Table 18-1).

References

1. Kim JE, Mantravadi, Hur EY, Covert DJ. Short-term intraocular pressure changes immediately after intravitreal injections of anti-vascular endothelial growth factor agents. *Am J Ophthalmol.* 2008;14 (6):930-934.
2. Rosenfeld PJ, Brown DM, Heier JS, et al. Ranibizumab for neovascular age-related macular degeneration. *N Engl J Med.* 2006;355(14):1419-1431.
3. Choi DY, Ortube MC, McCannel CA, et al. Sustained elevated intraocular pressures after intravitreal injection of bevacizumab, ranibizumab, and pegaptanib. *Retina.* 2011;31(6):1028-1035.
4. Hoang QV, Mendonca LS, Della Torre KE, et al. Effect on intraocular pressure in patients receiving unilateral intravitreal anti-vascular endothelial growth factor injections. *Ophthalmology.* 2012;119(2):321-326.

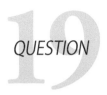

QUESTION

WHAT IS THE BEST WAY TO CLASSIFY
ANGLE CLOSURE GLAUCOMAS?

Anna K. Junk, MD

Angle closure describes appositional or synechial closure of the anterior chamber angle based on the presence of iridotrabecular contact (ITC) on gonioscopy. Therefore, gonioscopy is essential for the diagnosis of angle closure. I prefer a dark room and start with a 1-mm, narrow slit beam well away from the pupil. While the patient maintains gaze in primary position, I use high magnification to identify the termination of the corneal wedge, which marks the anterior edge of the trabecular meshwork (TM). To minimize distortion, I avoid tilting of the lens. It is essential to determine whether the angle is occludable, or in other words whether the iris is in contact with the TM. If there is no ITC, I estimate the geometric angle between the TM and adjacent peripheral iris. Once this has been completed for the entire circumference, I proceed to dynamic (indentation) gonioscopy. This will assess whether ITC is appositional or synechial (permanent). While Goldmann-style lenses can enhance the examiner's ability to identify important anatomical angle landmarks and pathology, the smaller diameter 4-mirror goniolenses are preferable for indentation. Anterior segment imaging devices may augment the angle evaluation (ultrasound biomicroscopy [UBM], anterior segment optical coherence tomography [OCT]). While 3 gonioscopic grading schemes are well known (Scheie, Shaffer, and Spaeth), a clear text description of the angle structures seen, angle width, iris contour, and amount of pigmentation is desirable.

The major demographic risk factors for primary angle closure are older age, female sex, and Asian ancestry. Ocular risk factors include narrower drainage angles, shallower axial and limbal anterior chamber depth, thicker lens, shorter axial length, more anteriorly positioned lens, smaller corneal diameter, and hypermetropic refraction. Historically, primary angle closure was classified into 3 subcategories based on symptoms: acute, subacute or intermittent, and chronic angle closure. Acute angle closure is associated with abrupt onset of symptomatic intraocular pressure (IOP) elevation as a result of total angle closure, which would typically not resolve by itself. Subacute angle closure describes a self-limiting and recurrent abrupt onset of symptomatic IOP rise

Gedde SJ, ed. *Curbside Consultation in Glaucoma:*
49 Clinical Questions, Second Edition (pp 89–90)
© 2015 Taylor & Francis Group

due to angle closure. Chronic angle closure is characterized by asymptomatic IOP elevation or posterior anterior synechiae (PAS) due to angle closure. While this classification is easy to understand for patients with symptoms, it does not consider risk for loss of visual function or offer guidance for management.

A new classification system for angle closure and angle closure glaucoma (ACG) was devised by the World Glaucoma Association consensus.[1] This classification scheme uses the anatomic level at which blockage occurs, the iris, the ciliary body, the lens, and vectors posterior to the lens. It facilitates understanding of the various mechanisms and treatment. There may be overlap, and treatment becomes more complex for each level of block.

- Level 1, iris and pupil: Pupillary block is the most common form of ACG. Aqueous flow is limited through the pupil in the region of iridolenticular contact. This creates a relative pressure gradient between the anterior and posterior chamber, causing anterior iris bowing, narrowing of the angle, and acute or chronic ITC or ACG.

- Laser peripheral iridotomy (LPI) eliminates the pressure differential between anterior and posterior chambers. The iris assumes a flatter configuration, and the iridocorneal angle widens. The iridolenticular contact increases as aqueous flows through the iridotomy.

- Level 2, ciliary body architecture: Also termed *plateau iris*, abnormal ciliary body position leads to angle closure when anteriorly positioned ciliary processes force the peripheral iris into the angle. On gonioscopy, the iris root may be short and insert anteriorly on the ciliary face, producing a shallow, narrow angle with a sharp drop-off of the peripheral iris. Laser iridotomy either fails to open the angle or opens it only partially. Iridoplasty may open the angle in these cases. Plateau iris syndrome refers to angle closure in eyes with plateau iris configuration despite the presence of a patent iridotomy. The angle can narrow further with age due to lens growth, and periodic gonioscopy is recommended. Rarely, iridociliary cysts, tumors, or ciliary body edema can mimic plateau iris configuration.

- Level 3, lens-induced glaucoma: Also known as *phacomorphic glaucoma*, anterior lens subluxation or intumescence may precipitate acute or chronic ACG due to the lens pressing against the iris and ciliary body and forcing them anteriorly.

- Level 4, ciliary block (malignant glaucoma, aqueous misdirection): Caused by forces posterior to the lens that push the lens-iris diaphragm forward, this condition presents the greatest diagnostic and treatment challenge of the ACGs. Swelling or anterior rotation of the ciliary body and relaxation of the zonular apparatus leads to anterior lens displacement, causing direct angle closure by physically pushing the iris against the TM. A shallow supraciliary detachment appears to cause the anterior rotation of the ciliary body but may not be evident on routine B-scan.

Other causes of angle closure: Anterior chamber processes causing PAS include iris and angle neovascularization, iridocorneal endothelial syndrome, and anterior uveitis. Other disease processes include anterior subluxation of the lens, iris or ciliary body cysts, ciliary body inflammation or tumor infiltration, and air or gas bubbles after intraocular surgery. These disorders should be identified and treated specifically.

Reference

1. Foster P, He M, Liebmann JM. *Epidemiology, Classification and Mechanism*. Vol Consensus Series. The Hague, the Netherlands: Kugler Publications; 2006.

SECTION III

GENERAL MANAGEMENT

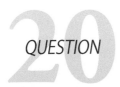

WHICH PATIENTS WITH OCULAR HYPERTENSION SHOULD I TREAT?

Husam Ansari, MD, PhD and
Richard K. Parrish II, MD

The Meaning of "Treatment"

Treatment is generally understood by patients to mean a medical or surgical intervention provided by doctors to either alleviate or prevent the signs and symptoms of a disease. From a practical standpoint, decisions within each individual patient-doctor relationship define the nature of the treatment. For example, although an internist may recommend medical therapy to an asymptomatic patient with several risk factors for developing ischemic heart disease, the patient determines whether the benefits of beginning treatment justify the possible risks and costs. A patient who does not wish to start medical therapy or modify his or her risk factors by stopping smoking, changing dietary habits, or beginning an exercise program may nonetheless desire to be monitored for the development of signs and symptoms of disease. Cardiac stress tests may be performed to determine whether asymptomatic disease has developed. The doctor who monitors these findings and symptoms provides patient care without initiating medical or surgical treatment.

Calculating the Global Risk of Developing Primary Open-Angle Glaucoma

Our decision regarding whether to begin medical therapy to lower intraocular pressure (IOP) in a patient with ocular hypertension (OHT) is comparable to determining whether to start treatment of an asymptomatic patient with risk factors for ischemic heart disease. The interaction

Gedde SJ, ed. *Curbside Consultation in Glaucoma:*
49 Clinical Questions, Second Edition (pp 93–96)
© 2015 Taylor & Francis Group

of several risk factors, such as elevated low-density lipoproteins, hypertension, a family history of myocardial infarction, and history of cigarette smoking, has been used to calculate a global risk of developing ischemic heart disease. The interaction of multiple factors has also been demonstrated to predict which groups of patients with OHT are more likely to develop primary open-angle glaucoma (POAG). The Ocular Hypertension Treatment Study (OHTS) and the European Glaucoma Prevention Study (EGPS) provided data on the conversion of OHT to POAG in 2 independent groups of patients that have been used to develop risk calculators.[1-4] The following risk factors have been used to calculate global risk for the conversion of OHT to POAG[4]:

- Age (years)—at current visit
- Baseline IOP (mm Hg)—average of the untreated IOP (of both eyes as determined over 3 visits within about 6 months)
- Central corneal thickness (microns)—average of 3 separate measurements from each eye at the same visit
- Pattern standard deviation (dB) (Humphrey Field Analyzer; Carl Zeiss Meditec, Jena, Germany)—average from 2 visual fields of each eye
- Vertical cup-to-disc ratio by contour—average of both eyes

The OHTS and EGPS risk calculators are available for use online at no charge and as an iPhone/iPad application ("OHT Calc") at a nominal price.[4]

So, All I Need Is a Good Risk Calculator, Right? Wrong!

Despite the development of validated risk calculators that provide estimates of global risk, we cannot definitively determine which individual patients would benefit most from IOP-lowering treatment. We need to consider several factors in addition to those entered into a risk calculator when deciding whether to begin IOP-lowering therapy (Table 20-1). These include life expectancy,[5] family history, ancestry, the status of the fellow eye, the presence or history of a disc hemorrhage,[6] and the safety, cost, and convenience of treatment. Although older age is positively associated with the development of POAG, the decision to treat older patients must take into account the shorter life expectancy in these patients. The lifelong risks of progression in a 55-year-old woman are likely greater than those of a 79-year-old patient, but the magnitude of the difference is not known. Also, current risk calculators are based on data from patients who were younger than 80 years at the time of enrollment in the OHTS and EGPS, so these studies cannot estimate the risk for patients beyond their eighth decade of life. Although family history and ancestry did not predict progression in a multivariate analysis in the OHTS, the increased risk of developing POAG in patients with first-degree relatives with POAG as well as in patients of African ancestry is well known. Therefore, family history and ancestry also inform our decision about whether to treat patients with OHT. In addition, we are more likely to treat a patient with OHT in one eye if the fellow eye has irreversible visual impairment from POAG or any other disease or if either eye has or has had a disc hemorrhage. Finally, a patient's risk tolerance and predisposition for or against treatment, as well as his or her ability to afford, tolerate, and comply with treatment, must be regarded in this decision. In many cases, an OHT patient with financial hardship or multiple drug allergies would benefit from regular monitoring without treatment.

Table 20-1
Patient Factors Favoring Treatment vs Observation in Ocular Hypertension

Factors Favoring Treatment	*Factors Favoring Observation*
Young age (longer life expectancy)	Older age (shorter life expectancy)
Older age (higher risk of POAG)	Younger age (lower risk of POAG)
Highly elevated untreated IOP	Borderline elevated untreated IOP
Thin central corneal thickness	Thick central corneal thickness
Increased vertical cup-to-disk ratio	Inability to afford treatment
Higher pattern standard deviation	Inability to tolerate treatment
Disc hemorrhage	Inability to comply with treatment
Positive family history	Patient preference against treatment
African ancestry	
POAG in fellow eye	
Poor vision in fellow eye (any cause)	
Low patient risk-tolerance	

Abbreviations: IOP, intraocular pressure; POAG, primary open-angle glaucoma.

What Are the Risks of Delaying IOP-Lowering Treatment?

The consequences of not treating patients with OHT who eventually convert to POAG are not known, although information is available on the natural history of early untreated POAG from the Early Manifest Glaucoma Trial.[7,8] It is not known if the rates of optic nerve and visual field change are constant in glaucoma, but it has been shown that treatment lowers these rates in patients with OHT.[9] Experimental animal studies in which severely elevated IOP is induced suggest that the rate of axonal loss and glaucomatous cupping may rapidly become exponential after initial injury has occurred.[10] In phase 2 of the OHTS,[11] patients in the observation group were offered treatment after 7.5 years of observation. Although there was no evidence of an increased incidence of POAG in the observation group even after the initiation of medication compared with the medication group, the data suggest that patients with OHT at high risk for developing POAG (> 13% risk by the OHTS/EPGS risk calculator) would benefit from more frequent observation and earlier treatment than would lower-risk patients.[11]

Summary

The decision to begin treatment of any asymptomatic condition cannot be made unless both the patient and the doctor perceive a genuine treatment benefit. Ultimately, the patient must decide not only when to begin treatment but whether to continue it. The emotional impact of factors that were not previously determined to affect the risk of conversion in a multivariate analysis of risk in patients with OHTS, such as a family history of POAG, cannot be ignored, particularly if this was associated with visual loss.

The most important decision that a patient and doctor will make is not to simply begin medical therapy but to commit to a long-standing relationship that will permit both to have the most complete information for making future decisions. From a practical standpoint, this means developing a doctor-patient relationship that understands both the value and limitations of our current global risk calculators and diagnostic tools.

References

1. Kass MA, Heuer DK, Higginbotham EJ, et al. The Ocular Hypertension Treatment Study: a randomized trial determines that topical ocular hypotensive medication delays or prevents the onset of primary open-angle glaucoma. *Arch Ophthalmol.* 2002;120:701-713.

2. Gordon MO, Beiser JA, Brandt JD, et al. The Ocular Hypertension Treatment Study: baseline factors that predict the onset of primary open-angle glaucoma. *Arch Ophthalmol.* 2002;120:714-720.

3. Ocular Hypertension Treatment Study Group: European Glaucoma Prevention Study Group, et al. Validated prediction model for the development of primary open-angle glaucoma in individuals in ocular hypertension. *Ophthalmology.* 2007;114:10-19.

4. Ocular Hypertension Treatment Study. Glaucoma risk estimator. http://ohts.wustl.edu/risk. Accessed February 23, 2014.

5. Griffin BA, Elliott MN, Coleman AL, et al. Incorporating mortality risk into estimates of 5-year glaucoma risk. *Am J Ophthalmol.* 2009;148:925-931.

6. Budenz DL, Anderson DR, Feuer WJ, et al. Detection and prognostic significance of optic disc hemorrhages during the Ocular Hypertension Treatment Study. *Ophthalmology.* 2006;113:2137-2143.

7. Heijl A, Leske MC, Bengtsson B, et al. Reduction of intraocular pressure and glaucoma progression: results from the Early Manifest Glaucoma Trial. *Arch Ophthalmol.* 2002;120:1268-1279.

8. Leske MC, Heijl A, Hussein M, et al. Factors for glaucoma progression and the effect of treatment: the Early Manifest Glaucoma Trial. *Arch Ophthalmol.* 2003;121:48-56.

9. De Moraes CG, Demirel S, Gardiner DK, et al. Effect of treatment on the rate of visual field change in the ocular hypertension treatment study observation group. *Invest Ophthalmol Vis Sci.* 2012;53:1704-1709.

10. Nickells R, Schlamp CL, Li Y, et al. Surgical lowering of elevated intraocular pressure in monkeys prevents progression of glaucomatous disease. *Exp Eye Res.* 2007;84:729-736.

11. Kass MA, Gordon MO, Gao F, et al. Delaying treatment of ocular hypertension: the Ocular Hypertension Treatment Study. *Arch Ophthalmol.* 2010;128:276-287.

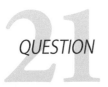
HOW SHOULD I SET A TARGET INTRAOCULAR PRESSURE?

Gregg A. Heatley, MD

It is tempting to immediately decide to treat all eyes with elevated intraocular pressure (IOP), but before you initiate treatment, stop and ask yourself what target to work toward. All eyes do not need the same IOP to be healthy. Your job is to determine the pressure this particular eye needs to minimize risk of progression (Figure 21-1).

How Much Room Do I Have to Be Wrong in Setting This Target?

If the situation is one of a dramatic loss of neural rim, thinning of the nerve fiber layer (NFL), and advanced visual field loss, you may only feel comfortable setting a target of "as low as possible" and choosing an absolute target irrespective of the starting IOP. In most clinical situations, when uveoscleral outflow is significantly less than conventional outflow, IOP can only go as low as episcleral venous pressure; therefore, "as low as possible" is 8 to 12 mm Hg, and the corresponding target is 12 mm Hg.

Is There Trustworthy, Reproducible Evidence of Damage?

If there is no evidence of damage and the IOP is high enough to convince you that there is a significant risk of future damage, then the Ocular Hypertension Treatment Study (OHTS) data

Gedde SJ, ed. *Curbside Consultation in Glaucoma:*
49 Clinical Questions, Second Edition (pp 97–100)
© 2015 Taylor & Francis Group

Figure 21-1. Flowchart for using clinical information to establish initial target pressure.

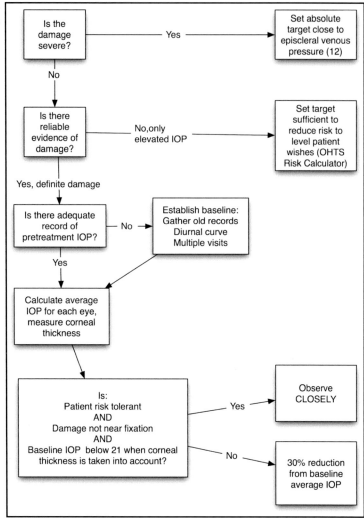

can help immensely to describe the likelihood of progression within 5 years. When I feel that the OHTS data are relevant, I will often take the patient to the website[1] or the grids and show the patient the relevant risk profile. Depending on the patient's risk tolerance/aversion, we may jointly set a fairly high or fairly low target. I have often been surprised by the answers from patients I thought I knew well enough that I could accurately predict their wishes. The step of intimately involving these patients in this choice pays huge dividends in compliance and understanding of the need for future follow-up visits.

Do I Know a Real Starting Point?

It is not uncommon for a glaucoma specialist to see a new patient who is referred for a single instance of elevated IOP measurement. In digging through the chart notes, I may or may not find many other IOP measurements, much less any others that are high. Daily variation in IOP is certainly great enough to result in a single measurement higher than the patient's typical range, and the practitioner choosing to treat should be sure that an adequate measure of this variability has been done. If old records are available, whether from another office or your own, make a point of transcribing them into the narrative of the note when the target is being established. In the absence of an IOP history, take the time to create one, with several visits over several days or, alternatively, a diurnal curve. The bare minimum is 3 trustworthy measurements.

What Artifacts Affect the Baseline and Target Intraocular Pressure Measurements?

The OHTS[2] was a landmark study for many reasons, from showing that lowering IOP really does reduce the risk of developing glaucoma damage to demonstrating that the cornea itself can be a major source of artifact in our IOP measurements. In the context of setting target pressure, the corneal thickness is less significant if the target is set as a percentage reduction from baseline but is definitely a factor if you are choosing an absolute number as a target. However, the pachymetry does come into play when making the choice of whether to follow or treat. If the patient has had mild damage and not near fixation, has "normal" IOP when corrected for corneal thickness, is tolerant of risk, and understands and agrees to the need for very close follow-up with frequent visual field testing, then you can choose to observe this patient closely and not treat until one of the variables should change (rise in IOP, progression of field or disc change, or the patient's feelings about risk change). Essentially, this means you have set a target pressure equal to the current IOP.

If Intraocular Pressure Lowering Is Needed, How Low Do I Need to Go?

The OHTS IOP-lowering goal was 20%, and this reduction was sufficient to reduce the odds of progressing (with very stringent thresholds) from about 10% to 5%. Most other studies have used a reduction of 30% as the treatment goal.[3,4] To my mind, a 30% reduction is intuitively great enough to have a definite, significant effect on the arc of the patient's glaucoma career, and I prefer to use that as my first and subsequent target adjustments. That is, if I have a good, reliable baseline IOP and reduce the IOP by 30%, and the patient then goes on to progress while at the first target IOP, I will reduce the target by another 30% and treat to achieve that reduction.

Should I Make a Goal of a Percentage Intraocular Pressure Drop or an Absolute Intraocular Pressure Target?

I prefer to use a straight percentage whenever possible. The useful side effect of using the percentage drop is that it self-adjusts for the effect of the corneal thickness on tonometry. If you were to use an absolute IOP target, extremely thin or thick corneas may make achieving that target effectively impossible or may result in far less IOP lowering than you wish.

Do I Know This Target Will Be Low Enough?

There is ample retrospective and prospective evidence to suggest that a 30% reduction will work for the average patient. Hopefully, in the not too distant future, we will be able to define a metric other than IOP or visual field testing that can be applied per patient, per eye that will give greater assurance of stopping glaucomatous progression. Whether this turns out to be an electrophysiologic or anatomic metric is anybody's guess, but there is definite hope that someday soon we will work to lower IOP in an individual eye until this metric shows that all the ganglion cells are healthy and then maintain that IOP for the life of the patient. Until then, the rule of 30% seems to be a very reasonable first approximation.

References

1. Washington University in St Louis School of Medicine. Glaucoma 5-year risk estimator. http://ohts.wustl.edu/risk/calculator.html. Accessed March 4, 1008.
2. Gordon MO, Beiser JA, Brandt JD, et al, for the Ocular Hypertension Treatment Study Group. The Ocular Hypertension Treatment Study: baseline factors that predict the onset of primary open-angle glaucoma. *Arch Ophthalmol.* 2002;120:714-720.
3. Schwartz, K, Budenz D. Current management of glaucoma. *Curr Opin Ophthalmol.* 2004;15:119-126.
4. Collaborative NTG Study Group. The effectiveness of IOP reduction in the treatment of NTG. *Am J Ophthalmol.* 1998;126:498-505.

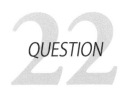

HOW SHOULD I BEGIN TREATMENT FOR A PATIENT WITH NEWLY DIAGNOSED PRIMARY OPEN-ANGLE GLAUCOMA?

Annisa L. Jamil, MD and
Richard P. Mills, MD, MPH

The diagnosis of primary open-angle glaucoma (POAG) carries with it different implications for the treating physician and the patient. For the physician, optimizing a treatment plan is a trial-and-error process often requiring several visits. For the patient, education about the chronic, asymptomatic nature of disease and techniques on how best to use the medication present unique challenges.

As clinicians, we know that establishing the diagnosis is often easier than planning and executing a treatment regimen. First, the degree of glaucomatous optic neuropathy and the concurrent damage to the visual field must be evaluated to set a target goal of intraocular pressure (IOP). It is important to recognize that once an optic disc has exhibited structural involvement, it is more susceptible to additional damage and may require lower target pressures. The previous chapter on establishing a target pressure highlights this important part of our treatment considerations. When we initiate therapy, we must have an open discussion with the patient about the chronic nature of disease that requires lifelong therapy. It may be a difficult concept to comprehend since many patients do not experience overt symptoms, other than those related to the side effects of topical medications used to treat their POAG. Education about this disease will help impart an awareness of the possible risk of irreversible blindness as well as establish the necessary steps to prevent it. Discussions should include a review of some of the pertinent clinical trials such as the Early Manifest Glaucoma Trial (EMGT), which clearly illustrates that with an average 25% decrease in baseline IOP, progression occurred in 45% of the treated patients compared with 62% in the untreated group.[1]

You should tailor the therapy for each patient to encourage adherence to the regimen. This requires taking into consideration many factors, including the patient's lifestyle, the financial burden, and the presence of other medical comorbidities. Some patients are self-aware and realize that persisting with a medical regimen is difficult, and therefore they may be ideal candidates for laser

Gedde SJ, ed. *Curbside Consultation in Glaucoma:
49 Clinical Questions, Second Edition* (pp 101–103)
© 2015 Taylor & Francis Group

trabeculoplasty. Also, for those with preexisting ocular surface disease, there are many preservative-free options that potentially will not exacerbate their underlying condition. Finally, patients must be informed about the potential side effects of each medication before initiating treatment.

For patients with early to moderate disease, topical medications or laser trabeculoplasty are reasonable options with comparable efficacy.[2] The goal of medical therapy is to control the pressure with the fewest medications and daily doses. A uniocular trial of medication is encouraged to verify an adequate decrease in IOP with the contralateral eye serving as a control. Although the uniocular trial may be confounded by a treatment response that is not always the same in both eyes, it is more often useful than not. Many patients may be using eye drops for the first time, so proper instillation techniques must be reviewed. Requiring the patients to demonstrate the technique in the clinic ensures that the medication has a good chance of getting into the eye. We schedule a 4-week return visit after initiating treatment to check whether the target pressure range is achieved. If there is minimal change in the IOP, we then inquire about problems with the use of the medication and, if there is none, the patient may be a nonresponder to the particular class of drops. In our practice, a prostaglandin analogue is initially tried because of its favorable side effect profile and the once-daily dosing schedule. If the initial medication is found to lower pressure but not to the desired target range, then additional medications may be necessary to provide adequate control. A β-blocker is a reasonable choice for additional therapy if there are no clear contraindications for use. When using topical therapy, it is essential to evaluate preexisting ocular surface disease because it is well established that patients with glaucoma have a higher degree of corneal staining.[3] Fortunately, more preservative-free medications are available for our patients that may provide long-term benefit without causing more issues for their underlying ocular surface disease.

Laser trabeculoplasty is a reasonable alternative for initial therapy in patients with an active lifestyle, those reluctant to take medications, or as an adjunct to existing medical therapy. It has an important role in the treatment of POAG that does not depend on patient adherence with a dosing schedule of topical medication. The Glaucoma Laser Trial demonstrated that within 2 years, eyes treated initially with argon laser trabeculoplasty (ALT) had better controlled IOP than those initially treated with timolol. In addition, after 7 to 9 years, the eyes treated first with ALT had a 1.2-mm Hg greater reduction in IOP than those treated with medication.[2] In our practice, selective laser trabeculoplasty has supplanted ALT because of the lack of tissue damage and comparable results, as well as theoretical repeatability.[4,5] Selective laser trabeculoplasty (SLT) has also been found to be as effective as latanoprost for initial management of POAG.[6] In our practice, we usually apply a 2-stage approach, treating 180 degrees at a time to minimize postoperative pressure spikes. Most patients respond well after the first stage, but if adequate pressure is not attained, there is always the possibility to treat the other half of the angle. Unfortunately, there is an attrition of efficacy experienced over time. Although trabeculoplasty does not guarantee a significant drop in IOP, it remains a viable option for patients who are intolerant to medications or would like to reduce the burden of topical therapy.

With the emerging field of glaucoma surgery, especially with the advent of minimally invasive glaucoma surgery (MIGS), there are many more potential surgical options for the primary treatment of open-angle glaucoma (OAG). Recently, it has been recognized that cataract extraction alone may decrease IOP, especially in patients with higher preoperative IOP.[7] For patients with early disease, there are also additional surgical options that can be done with or without cataract extraction such as the Trabectome (NeoMedix, Tustin, California) or the iStent (Glaukos, Laguna Hills, California). Trabeculectomy may be considered a primary treatment for some patients. Certainly, it has an absolute role in patients with severe disease where immediate IOP control is paramount; however, as first-line therapy for a newly diagnosed patient, it requires further deliberation. The Collaborative Initial Glaucoma Treatment Study (CIGTS) looked at patients randomized to 1 of 2 study arms: aggressive treatment with medications or initial trabeculectomy. At 5 years, they found similar results in IOP control with equalization of vision between the 2 groups (however,

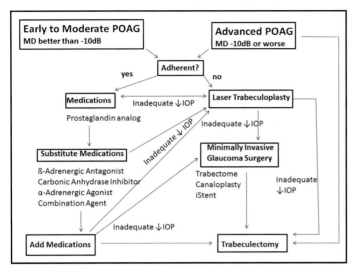

Figure 22-1. Treatment options for the management of POAG. (Reprinted with permission of Annisa L. Jamil, MD.)

surgery patients required more cataract surgery). More important, after 5 years, the visual field loss was comparable between the trabeculectomy and medication-only groups.[4] Although trabeculectomy clearly remains the gold standard for definitively lowering IOP, the benefits must outweigh the risks of hypotony, bleb leaks, dysesthesia, and infection. For that reason, our newly diagnosed patients with early to moderate disease are usually given a medication trial or laser trabeculoplasty before consideration of incisional surgery. In newly diagnosed patients with more advanced glaucoma (mean deviation, −10 dB or worse), consideration should be given to initial trabeculectomy based on reported findings from the CIGTS of better outcomes with surgery in this group of patients.[4] Please refer to Figure 22-1 for an illustration of treatment options for managing POAG.

There are many approaches to the treatment of our patients with newly diagnosed POAG. Thorough evaluation of each patient's optic nerve involvement and determination of adequate IOP control are keys to initiation of therapy. Attention to our patient's understanding and education of the disease further increases the likelihood of our success.

References

1. Heijl A, Leske AC, Bengtsson B, et al. Reduction of intraocular pressure and glaucoma progression: results from the Early Manifest Glaucoma Trial. *Arch Ophthalmol.* 2002;120:1268-1279.
2. The Glaucoma Laser Trial Research Group. The Glaucoma Laser Trial (GLT). 2. Results of argon laser trabeculoplasty versus topical medications. *Ophthalmology.* 1990;97:1403-1413.
3. Juzych MS, Chopra V, Banitt MR, et al. Comparison of long-term outcomes of selective laser trabeculoplasty versus argon laser trabeculoplasty in open-angle glaucoma. *Ophthalmology.* 2004;111:1853-1859.
4. Lichter PR, Musch DC, Gillespie BW, Guire KE, Janz NK, Wren PA, Mills RP. Interim clinical outcomes in the Collaborative Initial Glaucoma Treatment Study comparing initial treatment randomized to medication or surgery. *Ophthalmology.* 2001 Nov;108 (11):1943-1953.
5. Musch DC, Gillespie BW, Niziol LM, Lichter PR. Baseline factors associated with visual field progression during long-term treatment for newly diagnosed open-angle glaucoma. Paper presented at: Association for Research in Vision and Ophthalmology Annual Meeting; May 2, 2006 Fort Lauderdale, FL.
6. McIlraith I, Strasfeld M, Colev G, Hutnik CM. Selective laser trabeculoplasty as initial and adjunctive treatment for open-angle glaucoma. *J Glaucoma.* 2006 Apr;15(2):124-130.
7. Poley B, Lindstrom R, Samuelson T, Schulze R. Intraocular pressure reduction after phacoemulsification with intraocular lens implantation in glaucomatous and nonglaucomatous eyes: evaluation of a causal relationship between the natural lens and open-angle glaucoma. *J Cataract and Refractive Surg.* 2009;35:1946-1955.

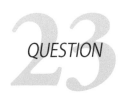
HOW SHOULD I MANAGE A PATIENT WHO IS PROGRESSING AT LOW LEVELS OF INTRAOCULAR PRESSURE?

Ta Chen Peter Chang, MD

When I see a patient with glaucoma who appears to be getting worse despite low pressures, the first thing I ask myself is whether the progression is real and whether there is an explanation other than glaucoma for the changes. Once I have confirmed the progression and ruled out the pressure-independent explanations, the next question is whether the pressure is really low—usually this is a question of adherence, but it can be a question of sampling error. Finally, I try to determine the rate of change so that I can balance the risks of advancing treatment against the risk of noticeable damage within the patient's lifetime (Figure 23-1). It has been suggested that in the context of age-related retinal ganglion cell deaths (5000 to 10,000 per year),[1] all glaucomatous diseases progress regardless of treatment.[2] Hence, the rate of disease progression is more important and clinically relevant than the question of whether progression occurs. Most of the time, the diagnostic and management dilemmas lie with progression that is thought to be more rapid and/or profound than would be expected based on the patient's intraocular pressure (IOP) level.

Question 1: Is the Progression "Real"?

Whenever structural or functional testing reveals possible progression, I confirm the finding before I change therapy. We know that this is especially important with regard to visual field testing, as evidenced by the results of the Collaborative Normal Tension Glaucoma Study.[3] In the Ocular Hypertension Treatment Study (OHTS), approximately 86% of abnormal visual fields were false positives upon retesting.[4] Some practices instruct their visual field technicians to repeat visual tests automatically on the same visit when the new test reveals possible glaucomatous progression from the patient's baseline.

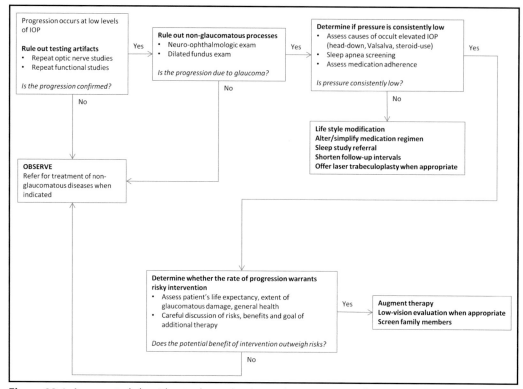

Figure 23-1. A suggested algorithm to the evaluation and management of a patient who is progressing at a low level of IOP.

Poor signal strength (≤6) on an optical coherence tomography (OCT) examination, which can result from media opacity or surface irregularity, can cause artifactual thinning of the circumpapillary retinal nerve fiber layer (RNFL).[5] Imaging technicians should be trained to pay close attention to the patients' ocular surface condition and apply ocular lubricants generously when indicated. They should also repeat tests several times if the image quality is poor.

Question 2: Is the Progression Related to Glaucoma?

Once testing artifact is ruled out, I perform a neuro-ophthalmologic and dilated fundus examination to look for a nonglaucomatous explanation for the patient's progression. Any concurrent decrease in visual acuity or color vision, the new onset of an afferent pupillary defect, or a finding of disc pallor out of proportion to cupping warrant neuro-ophthalmologic consultation. Similarly, any confirmed visual field progression in a young patient with truly low levels of IOP would warrant neuro-ophthalmologic consultation. Lesions such as a retinal vein or artery occlusion and/or an exudative macular pathology can introduce new paracentral and arcuate scotomata that mimic glaucomatous loss. Hence, I routinely perform a dilated fundus examination in the setting of new scotoma or the broadening of an existing scotoma to rule out retinal pathology.

Question 3: Is the Pressure Really Low?

If the patient has significant glaucomatous progression despite low IOP levels, I try to determine if the pressure is consistently low. Some causes of occult IOP elevation between visits would include any prolonged head-down positioning (eg, yoga), significant Valsalva maneuvers (eg, professional wind instrument player), or concurrent, intermittent use of corticosteroid medications. Furthermore, evidence is emerging linking obstructive sleep apnea (OSA) to glaucomatous optic neuropathy. Hence, I routinely screen and refer patients with OSA risk factors for formal evaluation. Finally, I check the central corneal thickness (CCT) in all patients as an IOP that may "seem" normal may actually be elevated if the CCT is very thin.

Most of the time, however, I do not find anything to support elevated pressure between visits other than possible nonadherence with treatment. Only about one-third of patients receiving chronic medical therapy are perfectly or near perfectly adherent to their medical regimen when tested with dosage monitors.[6] But a noncompliant patient who uses his or her medication before an office visit may demonstrate progression despite an apparently low IOP. Several factors have been shown to be linked to poor compliance with medication, including medication side effects, cost, polypharmacy, dosing inconvenience, and patients' misunderstanding of instructions. The more complicated the medication regimen, the more likely is poor adherence. The topic of medication compliance must be approached with an empathic and nonjudgmental tone. A careful discussion of medication dosage, side effect, cost, and the patient's general comfort level with medication use can be helpful in personalizing therapy for the patient. In general, by switching to generic substitutions, consolidating the number of medications, and reviewing dosing schedules with written instructions, compliance can be improved and progression slowed. In appropriate candidates, laser trabeculoplasty should be offered as means of IOP control without reliance on patient compliance.

When I am trying to come up with a workable medication regimen for a patient, I usually see him or her frequently. Assuming that compliance improves before a scheduled office visit, by simply shortening the follow-up interval, better compliance may be achieved. Frequent follow-up also helps to identify those patients whose glaucoma progresses at a dangerous rate despite optimized medical therapy.

Question 4: Does the Rate of Progression Warrant Risky Interventions?

All treatments carry risks. When a patient is getting worse, I try to determine if the rate of glaucomatous progression is likely to threaten my goal of preserving good vision for his or her lifetime. Glaucoma progression is particularly likely to have a negative impact on the quality of life of patients with advanced visual field loss, those with long life expectancies, or patients who are monocular or have severe disease in their fellow eye. On the other hand, modest progression in those of advanced age and/or poor health can be observed.

Question 5: What Are the Risks, Benefits, and Goals of Augmenting Therapy?

Some patients will not be able to adhere to a medication regimen that adequately controls their IOP. Others, despite frequent follow-up and improved medication compliance, will have rapid progression despite a truly low level of IOP. In these patients, incisional surgery may be indicated. The effect of any pressure-lowering therapy diminishes with the IOP level to which it is applied, while the side effect profiles remain unchanged. Hence, glaucoma surgery on an eye with low levels of IOP has a higher risk/benefit ratio than does surgery on a patient with elevated IOP. The decision of whether additional surgery is appropriate is individualized to each patient, with careful discussion of the risks, benefits, and realistic goals and expectations of each procedure. In cases of bilateral, high-risk progression, surgery can be offered first to one eye and then to the fellow eye once it is established that the first eye fared better after surgical intervention.[7]

Question 6: What Else Can I Offer?

In the end, there are patients who will progress to end-stage glaucoma despite the physician and patient's best collective efforts. It is important that the patient does not feel abandoned, even if the physician can offer nothing further therapeutically. A timely referral for low-vision evaluation can greatly improve the patient's quality of life, while reminders to screen family members for glaucoma may allow early detection and treatment in their diseases and thus improve outcome.

Acknowledgment

The author thanks Dr. Elizabeth Hodapp (Bascom Palmer Eye Institute, Miami, Florida) for her suggestion and guidance in the preparation of this chapter.

References

1. Frisen L. High pass resolution and age related loss of visual pathway neurons. *Acta Ophthalmol.* 1991;69:511-515.
2. Singh K. Is the patient getting worse? *Open Ophthalmol J.* 2009;3:65-66.
3. Collaborative Normal-Tension Glaucoma Study Group. Comparison of glaucomatous progression between untreated patients with normal-tension glaucoma and patients with therapeutically reduced intraocular pressures. *Am J Ophthalmol.* 1998;126(4):487-497.
4. Keltner JL, Johnson CA, Quigg JM, Cello KE, Kass MA, Gordon MO, for the Ocular Hypertension Study Group. Confirmation of visual field abnormalities in the Ocular Hypertension Treatment Study. *Arch Ophthalmol.* 2000;118:1187-1194.
5. Wu Z, Huang J, Dustin L, Sadda SR. Signal strength is an important determinant of accuracy of nerve fiber layer thickness measurement by optical coherence tomography. *J Glaucoma.* 2009;18(3):213-216.
6. Budenz DL. A clinician's guide to the assessment and management of nonadherence in glaucoma. *Ophthalmology.* 2009;116(11)(suppl):S43-S47.
7. Hodapp E, Parrish RK, Anderson DR. *Clinical Decisions in Glaucoma.* St Louis, MO: Mosby-Year Book; 1993.

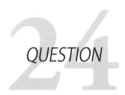

ARE THERE SPECIAL ISSUES OF WHICH I SHOULD BE AWARE REGARDING PIGMENT DISPERSION SYNDROME OR PIGMENTARY GLAUCOMA?

Celso Tello, MD; Sung Chul Park, MD; and
Robert Ritch, MD

Pigment dispersion syndrome (PDS) and pigmentary glaucoma (PG) are 2 successive stages of the same disease process characterized by disruption of the iris pigment epithelium (IPE) and deposition of the dispersed pigment granules throughout the anterior segment. The underlying anatomic cause of PDS is the presence of an iris concavity that allows apposition of its posterior surface to the zonular apparatus during pupillary movement or, to a greater degree, accommodation. The underlying etiology of the iris concavity remains unclear. Campbell and others[1-2] hypothesized that a reverse pupillary-block mechanism exists in which the iris drapes over the lens and acts as a "flap valve," preventing aqueous in the anterior chamber from returning to the posterior chamber. The pressure in the anterior chamber then exceeds that of the posterior chamber, pushing the iris posteriorly and creating a concave configuration, and forces the IPE into contact with the zonular bundles. Friction during pupillary movement disrupts the IPE, releasing pigment granules into the aqueous humor. The greater the contact, the greater the pigment dispersion should be.

The classic diagnostic triad that characterizes PDS consists of pigment deposits on the corneal endothelium (Krukenberg's spindle) (Figure 24-1); slit-like, radial, mid-peripheral iris transillumination defects (Figure 24-2); and dense homogeneous pigmentation of the trabecular meshwork (TM) (Figure 24-3). In PDS, the anterior chamber is deeper both centrally and peripherally. The angle is typically wide open, the iris is inserted posteriorly on the ciliary body, and the configuration of the peripheral iris is concave (Figure 24-4).

Patients can also present with iris heterochromia due to deposition of pigment particles on the iris surface when the involvement is asymmetric. Pigment may also be deposited on Schwalbe's line, the zonules, the posterior capsule of the lens at the level of the insertion of the posterior zonular fibers (Zentmayer ring), and the posterior lens central to Weigert's ligament (Scheie stripe).

Gedde SJ, ed. *Curbside Consultation in Glaucoma:*
49 Clinical Questions, Second Edition (pp 109–113)
© 2015 Taylor & Francis Group

Figure 24-1. PDS with Krukenberg's spindle.

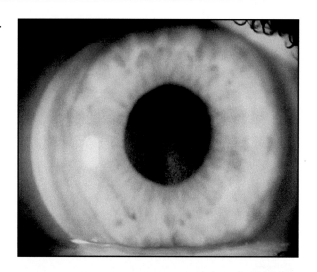

Figure 24-2. Mid-peripheral, radial, slit-like pattern transillumination defects are seen most commonly inferonasally in young patients with PDS/PG.

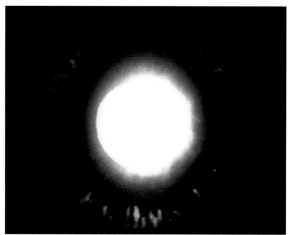

Figure 24-3. In PDS, the angle is characteristically wide open, with a homogeneous, dense hyperpigmented band on the trabecular meshwork. The iris insertion is posterior and the peripheral iris approach is often concave.

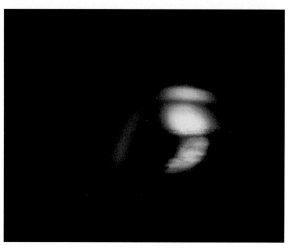

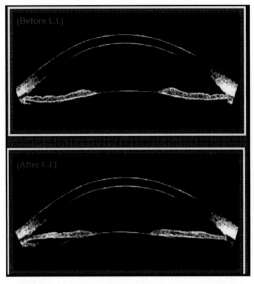

Figure 24-4. Ultrasound biomicroscopy demonstrates iris concavity (top) and iris flattening after laser iridotomy in a young patient with PDS (bottom).

As a result of obstruction of the inter-TM space by pigment granules and possible failure or breakdown of normal phagocytic function of trabecular endothelial cells, the intraocular pressure (IOP) elevates in many patients with PDS. The frequency with which PDS converts to PG has probably been greatly overestimated. The 3 studies that have examined patients longitudinally suggest that up to 50% will eventually develop PG.[3-5] However, the true rate of PDS in the general population may be an order of magnitude greater than has previously been suspected. We think that the true rate of progression to glaucoma is on the order of 10%.

PDS is an autosomal dominant disorder. The most significant risk factors for the development of the phenotypic expressions of PDS are young age, male sex, myopia, European ancestry, and a positive family history. Although men and women are equally affected, men are more likely to develop glaucoma at a ratio of approximately 3:1. PDS is typically bilateral and symmetric, although asymmetry may occur because a second condition exists, such as exfoliation syndrome, angle recession, and cataract formation or extraction.

Active release of pigment usually occurs during the second to fourth decade of life, when accommodation may play a significant role in the mechanism of the disease. The fact that accommodation increases iris concavity not only in patients with PDS but also in myopes without PDS and normal eyes suggests that the iris in PDS, in addition to being morphologically larger and concave, may be naturally predisposed to release its pigment. Loss of accommodation with the onset of presbyopia and development of relative pupillary block secondary to increased lens thickness with age presumably contribute to the cessation of pigment liberation and decrease the severity of PDS in middle age. With time, the transillumination defects may disappear, the IOP may return to normal, and the TM pigmentation may clear and become darker superiorly vs inferiorly ("pigment reversal sign").

Exercise (jogging, basketball, and bouncing during dancing) can cause release of a larger amount of pigment as a result of pupillary movements in young patients with PDS. This phenomenon can be prevented by miotic-induced pupillary block. Laser iridotomy to flatten the iris incompletely inhibits exercise-induced pigment release.

Other disorders that cause anterior segment pigment dispersion include exfoliation syndrome, iris pigment epithelial cysts, ciliary body cysts, iris nevus, and melanomas of the anterior or posterior segment; however, these conditions will not have a typical Krukenberg's spindle or the transillumination defects seen in PDS. Pigmented long anterior zonule syndrome (PLAZ) is an uncommon disorder that occurs when abnormally long and anteriorly inserted zonules are present on the face of the anterior lens capsule, usually bilaterally. These zonules rub against the posterior surface of the iris, liberating pigment into the anterior chamber. Krukenberg's spindles, densely pigmented TM, and pigmented zonules may be seen on examination. Iris transillumination defects are not typically found in PLAZ, nor is there reverse pupillary block. Unlike PDS, PLAZ incidence increases with hyperopia and age and in females. Finally, PLAZ is in some cases associated with a *CTRP5* genetic mutation and late-onset macular degeneration.

The treatment of PDS/PG is based on lowering IOP and preventing pigment release by reversing the iris concavity. Once the IOP is elevated, we prefer to treat with prostaglandin analogues that produce an excellent IOP response by increasing uveoscleral outflow. On the other hand, agents that lower IOP by reducing aqueous production may diminish the rate of clearance of the pigment from the TM and possibly exacerbate the disease process.

Theoretically, miotics are ideal drugs to reduce IOP in PDS/PG. Pupillary constriction reverses the iris concavity and eliminates iridozonular contact (inhibiting pigment release), and by creating tension over the scleral spur, miotics facilitate aqueous outflow through the TM, lower IOP, and enhance clearance of pigment. In patients with iris concavity and active release of pigment, low-concentration pilocarpine can be used as tolerated. The peripheral retina should be examined carefully prior to treatment with miotics since lattice degeneration is commonly found in myopes with PDS, and the incidence of retinal detachment is approximately 6% to 8%.

Argon laser trabeculoplasty (ALT) and selective laser trabeculoplasty are alternative treatments to lower IOP mostly in young pigmentary patients. The success rate of ALT in PG is greater in younger patients than in older ones and decreases with age. Selective laser trabeculoplasty should be performed with low energy to avoid release of pigment and resultant IOP spikes.

Laser iridotomy, by equalizing pressures between the anterior chamber (AC) and posterior chamber (PC), flattens the iris, eliminates iris-zonular contact, and prevents further liberation of pigment. Who should undergo laser iridotomy? Ostensibly, by preventing pigment liberation from the iris, the TM would have time to clear itself of pigment already deposited and reduce or eliminate further deposition. Therefore, only patients who are in the active stage of pigment liberation are good candidates. If pigment is liberated into the anterior chamber with pupillary dilation or exercise, it is suggestive that the patient is still in this stage. Patients who have uncontrolled glaucoma and are facing surgery are not ideal candidates for laser iridotomy. Although the benefits of laser iridotomy in PDS are inconclusive, laser iridotomy in young patients with iris concavity and active release of pigment (pigment liberation after dilation or after exercise) but without ocular hypertension or PG may provide a benefit for years. A prospective, randomized clinical trial by Scott et al[6] reported that there was no benefit of Nd:YAG laser iridotomy in preventing conversion from PDS with ocular hypertension (IOP >21 mm Hg) to PG. They postulated that laser iridotomy may be ineffective at a later stage with an elevated IOP and a damaged trabecular meshwork but may be effective in patients with minimal trabecular meshwork damage and no ocular hypertension.

References

1. Campbell DG. Pigmentary dispersion and glaucoma: a new theory. *Arch Ophthalmol.* 1979;97:1667-1672.
2. Campbell DG, Schertzer RM. Pigmentary glaucoma. In: Ritch R, Shields MB, Krupin T, eds. *The Glaucomas.* 2nd ed. St Louis, MO: CV Mosby; 1996:975-991.
3. Farrar SM, Shields MB, Miller KN, Stoup CM. Risk factors for the development and severity of glaucoma in the pigment dispersion syndrome. *Am J Ophthalmol.* 1989;108:223-229.
4. Migliazzo CV, Shaffer RN, Nykin R, Magee S. Long-term analysis of pigmentary dispersion syndrome and pigmentary glaucoma. *Ophthalmology.* 1986;93:1528-1536.

5. Richter CU, Richardson TM, Grant WM. Pigmentary dispersion syndrome and pigmentary glaucoma. A prospective study of the natural history. *Arch Ophthalmol.* 1986;104:211-215.

6. Scott A, Kotecha A, Bunce C, et al. YAG laser peripheral iridotomy for the prevention of pigment dispersion glaucoma: a prospective, randomized, controlled trial. *Ophthalmology.* 2011;118:468-473.

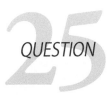

QUESTION 25

Does Exfoliation Syndrome Increase the Risk of Developing Glaucoma?

Are Patients With Exfoliation Glaucoma More Likely to Progress?

What Other Issues Do These Patients Have?

Robert Ritch, MD

Exfoliation syndrome (XFS) is a genetically determined age-related disease of elastic fibers characterized by the excessive production and progressive accumulation of a fibrillogranular extracellular material in many ocular and extra-ocular tissues. It is the most common identifiable cause of open-angle glaucoma (OAG) worldwide, comprising the majority of glaucoma in some countries.[1] It is diagnosed on slit-lamp examination by visualization of a characteristic pattern of whitish material on the anterior lens surface and often on the pupillary border of the iris (Figure 25-1). The diagnosis should be suspected in the absence of exfoliation material when various signs related to disruption of the iris pigment epithelium and pigment dispersal throughout the anterior chamber are present, which define patients as "exfoliation suspects." These include loss of the pigment ruff, iris transillumination defects adjacent to the pupil border, and increased trabecular pigment (Figures 25-2 and 25-3). It has been estimated that approximately 80 million people in the world have XFS. About 25% develop elevated intraocular pressure (IOP), and of these, one-third (ie, 6 to 7 million people) have glaucoma.

The prognosis of exfoliation glaucoma is worse than that of primary open-angle glaucoma (POAG), with higher mean IOP and greater frequency and severity of optic nerve and visual field damage at the time of diagnosis, greater diurnal fluctuation, poorer response to medications, more severe clinical course, and more frequent necessity for surgical intervention.[1] Patients with XFS develop elevated IOP at approximately 6 times the rate of patients without XFS. In the Early Manifest Glaucoma Trial (EMGT), XFS was the most significant correlate with progression of glaucoma, doubling the chance.

Involvement of the iris, lens, and blood vessels leads to anterior segment hypoxia, chronic blood-aqueous barrier breakdown, cataract, and abnormalities of ocular blood flow. Fragmentation of the zonular apparatus is an integral part of XFS, leading to lens laxity, anterior lens movement, and perhaps weakness of the lens capsule, while the pupils in these eyes dilate poorly, leading both

Gedde SJ, ed. *Curbside Consultation in Glaucoma:*
49 Clinical Questions, Second Edition (pp 115–118)

Figure 25-1. An early stage of XFS with cleft formation secondary to iridolenticular rubbing. The advanced, classic 3-ring appearance is known, but this is the stage at which it is important to make the diagnosis because it usually occurs prior to the development of glaucoma, which is potentially preventable.

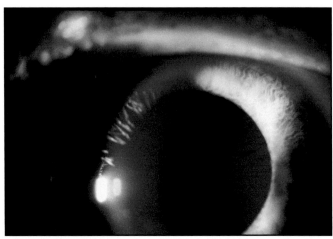

Figure 25-2. Typical iridocorneal angle appearance in an eye with XFS. The presence of spotty pigment on Schwalbe's line and a wavy Sampaolesi line should prompt the examiner to look carefully for XFS.

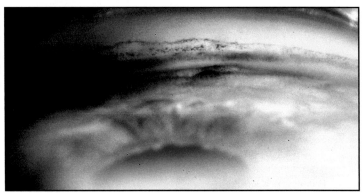

Figure 25-3. Loss of the iris pigment ruff should be another tip-off to the examiner to look carefully for XFS, particularly if it is unilateral or asymmetric.

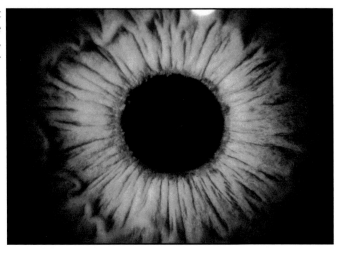

to increased intraoperative complications at the time of cataract extraction, such as zonular dialysis, capsular rupture, vitreous loss, and retained lens fragments, and to postoperative difficulties, such as chronic low-grade inflammation, intraocular lens decentration and subluxation, corneal endothelial decompensation, posterior capsular opacification, and capsular contraction syndrome.[1]

The prevalence of XFS varies among ethnic groups and races, and although the discovery of 2 nonsynonymous single-nucleotide polymorphisms (SNPs) in the *LOXL1* (lysyl oxidase-like 1) gene accounts for the vast majority of cases of the disease, not all persons homozygous for these SNPs develop the disease and not all persons with XFS develop glaucoma. Other factors, such as modifier genes, epigenetic factors, oxidative stress and inflammation, and environmental and dietary factors (eg, caffeine and folic acid consumption and diets high in antioxidants) are under investigation.

XFS is not just a disease of the eye, and deposits of fibrillogranular material resembling exfoliation material (although perhaps not precisely identical at a biochemical level) can be found in blood vessels, extraocular tissues, and diverse organs throughout the body.[2] Increasingly noted associations with systemic and central nervous system abnormalities elevate this disorder from not only a leading cause of glaucoma but to a condition of potential general widespread medical importance. Associations have been reported with transient ischemic attacks, stroke, myocardial ischemia and infarction, cerebrovascular insufficiency, Alzheimer disease, hearing loss, and hyperhomocysteinemia. Unfortunately, the correct diagnosis is often overlooked and its ramifications unrealized.

XFS is a cause of both open-angle and angle closure glaucoma and is etiologically associated with cataract formation and retinal vein occlusion. Decreased ascorbic acid in the anterior chamber in eyes with XFS may result in oxidative damage to the lens. The exfoliation material is rubbed off the surface of the lens by the iris and is deposited primarily in the trabecular meshwork. At the same time, the material on the surface of the lens acts like sandpaper during iridozonular friction and causes disruption of the iris pigment epithelium, liberating pigment particles from the iris sphincter region. These are dispersed throughout the anterior segment. This change is reflected in iris sphincter region transillumination, loss of the pupillary ruff, increased trabecular pigmentation, and pigment deposition on the iris surface.[3]

Exfoliative glaucoma responds less well to medical therapy than does POAG. The stepwise approach to its management is nonetheless similar to POAG and includes β-adrenergic antagonists, α-adrenergic agonists, miotics, prostaglandin analogues, carbonic anhydrase inhibitors, and laser and intraocular surgery.[4] Response to these interventions, however, differs compared to patients with POAG.

The fact that two-thirds of patients present with unilateral disease (although exfoliation material can be found on electron microscopy of the conjunctiva and iris of the fellow eye) and that about 50% develop involvement in 15 years has been long noted but its potential importance overlooked. The discovery of what genetic, immune, or other factors prevent or retard the development of XFS in the fellow eye may eventually shed light on a way to prevent the development of this unique and long underinvestigated disease.

Theoretically, miotics should be the first line of treatment. Not only do they lower IOP, but they should enable the meshwork to clear more rapidly by increasing aqueous outflow and should slow the progression of the disease by limiting pupillary movement, whereas treatment with aqueous suppressants may worsen trabecular function and iridolenticular friction.[3] Restriction of pupillary movement can lead to undisturbed buildup of exfoliation material. Pilocarpine 2% every night at bedtime not only increases aqueous outflow but interferes with the mechanism of development of the disease, providing an approximately 3-mm nonreactive pupil and minimizing release of exfoliation material from the lens and iris pigment by inhibiting iridolenticular friction. A prostaglandin analogue is my next drug since these drugs increase uveoscleral outflow. I use aqueous suppressants only after these have failed.

Argon laser trabeculoplasty (ALT) is particularly effective, at least early on, in eyes with XFS. The baseline IOP is usually higher than in eyes with POAG undergoing ALT, and the initial drop in IOP is greater. The increased effectiveness may be related to the increased trabecular pigmentation in XFS. Long-term success drops to approximately 35% to 55% at 3 to 6 years. Approximately 20% of patients develop sudden, late rises of IOP within the first 2 years after treatment. Continued pigment liberation may overwhelm the restored functional capacity of the meshwork, and maintenance miotic therapy to minimize papillary movement after ALT might counteract this. Selective laser trabeculoplasty (SLT) has been reported to be equally effective in lowering IOP in eyes with XFS. At the present time, since SLT is repeatable and ALT can be applied only once over the 360 degrees of the trabecular meshwork, it seems reasonable to initiate therapy with SLT and, if that is unsuccessful, then proceed to ALT. The results of trabeculectomy are comparable to those in POAG. Trabectome and tube shunt surgery are also viable surgical options.

References

1. Ritch R, Schlötzer-Schrehardt U. Exfoliation syndrome. *Surv Ophthalmol.* 2001;45:265-315.
2. Schlötzer-Schrehardt U, Naumann GOH. Ocular and systemic pseudoexfoliation syndrome. *Am J Ophthalmol.* 2006;141:921-937.
3. Ritch R, Schlötzer-Schrehardt U, Konstas AGP. Why does glaucoma occur in exfoliation syndrome? *Prog Retinal Eye Res.* 2003;22:253-275.
4. Konstas AGP, Tsironi S, Ritch R. Current concepts in the pathogenesis and management of exfoliation syndrome. *Compr Ophthalmol Update.* 2006;7:131-141.

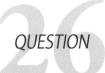
HOW FREQUENT IS
CORTICOSTEROID-INDUCED GLAUCOMA?
HOW SHOULD I MANAGE IT?

Davinder S. Grover, MD, MPH and
Alan L. Robin, MD

We have known for almost half a century that the use of both systemic and ocular corticosteroids can lead to an elevation of intraocular pressure (IOP). The IOP elevation is related to the type of corticosteroid and concentration, as well as route, frequency, and duration of administration. Usually, we are unable to stop corticosteroid treatment for a condition that is vision threatening. This chapter discusses the mechanism of IOP elevation, dose relationship between IOP elevation and corticosteroids, time course of response, risk factors, patient monitoring strategies, and treatment recommendations.

Although the exact mechanism is not known, we are fairly confident that the basic pathophysiology involves outflow obstruction rather than increased aqueous production. Many mechanisms have been proposed such as direct activation of corticosteroid receptors on specific cells in the trabecular meshwork, particulate matter deposited in the trabecular meshwork that can be observed gonioscopically, and inhibition of the production of outflow-enhancing prostaglandins.[1] We have seen an accumulation of glycosaminoglycans caused presumably by inhibiting the degradation of extracellular matrix material within the trabecular meshwork.[2–4]

With an increasing use of injectable corticosteroids in ophthalmology (intravitreal and periocular), there appears to be a marked increase in the observed frequency of corticosteroid-induced IOP elevation. Thankfully, one study found that even though almost half of patients might have IOPs over 21 mm Hg, most are responsive to topical and systemic IOP-lowering medications.[5] Although relatively unusual, marked IOP elevations associated with intravitreal use have been reported to occur as soon as 4 days after injection.[6] Less than 5% have IOPs over 40 mm Hg or undergo filtering surgery for IOP reduction. After an IOP elevation associated with topical corticosteroids, the IOP usually returns to normal within 1 to 3 weeks.[7] Complications from injectable corticosteroids are more difficult to treat than those from topical corticosteroids, as you can merely stop taking eye drops.

Gedde SJ, ed. *Curbside Consultation in Glaucoma:*
49 Clinical Questions, Second Edition (pp 119–121)
© 2015 Taylor & Francis Group

Previous studies have demonstrated that there is a dose-dependent relationship between corticosteroid use and IOP elevation.[1] Interestingly, the route of administration can also affect the degree and time course of IOP elevation. For example, 4 to 6 weeks following topical administration of corticosteroids, 5% of the population demonstrated a rise in IOP of more than 16 mm Hg and 30% demonstrated a rise of 6 to 15 mm Hg.[8] In another study, patients who received intravitreal administration of triamcinolone acetonide demonstrated a rise in IOP within 1 week. Also, an IOP rise of more than 10 mm Hg was detected in 22% of patients, and an IOP rise of more than 15 mm Hg was detected in 11% of patients.[5] The clinically challenging aspects of corticosteroid-induced glaucoma are determining not only the variability in responsiveness among patients and the variability in administration but also whether the corticosteroid or the underlying disease process (eg, uveitis) is causing the IOP elevation.

Fortunately, certain risk factors can be used to guide clinical practice and decision making. Studies have demonstrated that preexisting glaucoma, a family history of glaucoma, younger age, frequency of injection, amount of injection, and baseline IOP > 15 mm Hg are all risk factors for a larger rise in IOP after treatment.[1,9] Most of these studies were retrospective and had highly variable selection criteria, follow-up, dose of injection, conclusions, and definitions of IOP elevation. Although our ability to extrapolate definitive conclusions from these studies is somewhat limited, we can use these studies to help direct our clinical decision making.

We can offer several recommendations to help ensure that our patients are closely monitored and treated appropriately in the setting of a corticosteroid-induced IOP rise. In our baseline assessment, we should document a history of glaucoma, prior intraocular surgeries, gonioscopy, an IOP, and the appearance of both the optic nerve head and the retinal nerve fiber layer (RNFL). On the basis of the time course of IOP elevation elucidated by previous studies, we recommend that patients have their IOP measured within the first 2 weeks after initiating corticosteroid therapy and then monthly for several months.[5] If an IOP rise occurs, treatment should be dictated by the clinical appearance of the optic nerve and visual field, as well as the degree of IOP elevation. Keep in mind that accurate and reliable perimetry is often difficult to perform because of associated macular pathology or extensive inflammation causing reduced vision. Usually glaucoma is a slowly progressive disease, but there are scant data on the rate of progression with those whose baseline IOPs might have been in the teens and then experience a prolonged IOP elevation greater than 45 mm Hg.

Topical IOP-lowering medications are very effective but should be patient specific. In patients with cystoid macular edema, we try to avoid prostaglandin analogues due to their possible association with macular edema. There is no perfect answer regarding at which IOP level therapy should be instituted. The results of the Ocular Hypertensive Treatment Study (OHTS) might not apply to this group of potentially more susceptible eyes whose experience with elevated IOP might have been relatively short.

Although various authors have quoted different proportions of patients undergoing surgical intervention for IOP reduction, most groups reported a low percentage of patients in whom surgery was necessary or performed. In one study,[5] topical glaucoma medications were used in patients whose IOP exceeded 25 mm Hg, and incisional surgery was performed if IOP continued to exceed 40 mm Hg despite maximum medical therapy or if progressive glaucomatous damage was observed. With this protocol, only 1% of eyes underwent surgical intervention. This study demonstrates both the need to monitor patients closely as well as the high likelihood that topical medications can sufficiently manage most cases of corticosteroid-induced IOP elevation.

If more aggressive intervention is needed, there are a few surgical options. Laser trabeculoplasty can be attempted, although there is limited evidence to support this treatment modality.[10,11] Either filtering surgery or an aqueous shunt is the next suitable step. One's intervention should be guided by the degree of preexisting glaucoma damage (if any), how well the glaucoma was controlled prior to the intravitreal injection, and the state of the conjunctiva. If there has been no prior intraocular surgery or if there was only cataract surgery with either a small scleral shelf or a clear corneal incision, a trabeculectomy is typically the better option. Alternatively, if more extensive surgery has been performed in the past, an aqueous shunt is usually indicated. In the setting of multiple prior failed glaucoma operations, an external cilioablative procedure is probably indicated. If there is a history of poorly controlled IOP in the setting of advanced glaucoma, a trabeculectomy with mitomycin C should probably be attempted to achieve the lowest postoperative IOP. There is a paucity of data on the efficacy of newer glaucoma procedures in eyes with corticosteroid-induced glaucoma.

There have been rare cases in the literature of patients who have had recalcitrant IOP elevation following periocular corticosteroid injections that only resolved following removal of the whitish plaque of residual corticosteroid; these cases have not been widely reported and are likely the exception rather than the rule. Removal of intravitreal triamcinolone is almost never recommended.

Summary

Corticosteroid use in ophthalmology is increasing given its therapeutic benefits in various forms of macular edema, intraocular neovascularization, and ocular inflammation. Although corticosteroid-induced IOP elevation may be a serious complication, with appropriate monitoring and appropriate IOP control (usually only with topical ocular hypotensive medications), the risk of glaucomatous damage can be mitigated in most patients, and the full benefit of ocular corticosteroids can be realized.

References

1. Jampol LM, Yannuzzi LA, Weinreb RN. Editorial: glaucoma and intravitreal steroids. *Ophthalmology*. 2005;112:948.
2. Renfro L, Snow JS. Ocular effects of topical and systemic steroids. *Dermatol Clin*. 1992;10:505-510.
3. Spaeth GL, Rodriguez MM, Weinreb S. Steroid-induced glaucoma: A. Persistent elevation of intraocular pressure. B. Histopathological aspects. *Trans Am Ophthalmol Soc*. 1977;75:353-381.
4. Wordinger RJ, Clark AF. Effects of glucocorticoids on the trabecular meshwork: towards a better understanding of glaucoma. *Prog Retina Eye Res*. 1999;18:629-667.
5. Jonas JB, Degenring RF, Kreissig I, Akkoyun I, Kamppeter BA. Intraocular pressure elevation after intravitreal triamcinolone acetonide injection. *Ophthalmology*. 2005;112:593-598.
6. Singh IP, Ahmad SI, Yeh D, et al. Early rapid rise in intraocular pressure after intravitreal triamcinolone acetonide injection. *Am J Ophthalmol*. 2004;138(2):286-287.
7. LeBlanc RP, Steward RH, Becker B. Corticosteroid provocative testing. *Invest Ophthalmol*. 1970;9:946-948.
8. Becker B. Intraocular pressure response to topical corticosteroids. *Invest Ophthalmol*. 1965;4:198-205.
9. Rhee DJ, Peck RE, Belmont J, et al. Intraocular pressure alterations following intravitreal triamcinolone acetonide. *Br J Ophthalmol*. 2006;90:999-1003.
10. Baser E, Seymenoglu R. Selective laser trabeculoplasty for the treatment of intraocular pressure elevation after intravitreal triamcinolone injection. *Can J Ophthalmol*. 2009;44:e21.
11. Rubin B, Taglienti A, Rothman RF, et al. The effect of selective laser trabeculoplasty on intraocular pressure in patients with intravitreal steroid-induced elevated intraocular pressure. *J Glaucoma*. 2008;17(4):287-292.

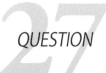
WHAT METHODS ARE AVAILABLE TO BREAK AN ACUTE ATTACK OF ANGLE CLOSURE GLAUCOMA?

Darrell WuDunn, MD, PhD

An acute angle closure glaucoma attack is one of the few true ophthalmic emergencies. Presenting symptoms include severe eye pain or pressure sensation, redness, blurred vision, seeing haloes around lights, and nausea/vomiting. Sometimes, the person will describe prior milder episodes of these symptoms in the affected or fellow eye. The examination reveals conjunctival hyperemia, microcystic corneal edema, a shallow peripheral anterior chamber, and a nonreactive, mid-dilated pupil. If the corneal edema is not too severe, you may see anterior chamber cells and optic disc swelling. Intraocular pressure (IOP) is usually very high (> 40 mm Hg). On gonioscopy of the involved eye, the angle is closed but indentation may open the angle in some areas; in the contralateral eye, the angle is usually narrow or appositionally closed, particularly superiorly, and peripheral anterior synechiae may be present.

Although pupillary block is the most common form of acute angle closure attack, you should also consider other conditions, especially with bilateral involvement or recent intraocular surgery. A medication history may reveal a recent addition or change in dose of topiramate or other sulfa compound or antidepressant. A myopic shift in the patient's refraction may also be found. The treatment of topiramate-induced angle closure attack is different from the treatment for pupillary block and is discussed in the last paragraph.

Attempts to lower IOP should be started promptly after the diagnosis is made because the acute pressure elevation can cause significant optic nerve damage within hours. Although laser iridotomy is the definitive treatment for acute, pupillary-block, angle closure glaucoma,[1] corneal edema may impair visualization. It is often very difficult to perforate the inflamed, edematous iris during an acute attack. Thus, immediate treatment should begin with corneal compression and medical therapy.

Corneal compression can be successful in some cases early in the attack. You may be able to see the angle open up with indentation gonioscopy. You should push the gonioprism posteriorly into

Gedde SJ, ed. Curbside Consultation in Glaucoma:
49 Clinical Questions, Second Edition (pp 123–126)
© 2015 Taylor & Francis Group

the central cornea and toward the mirror you are looking into so that the peripheral cornea vaults over the visible angle. This increases the chamber angle in the viewing quadrant. You can also indent the cornea with a moistened cotton-tip applicator. Note that the corneal epithelium is often edematous and prone to sloughing off with corneal compression and gonioscopy. Try these maneuvers for 30 seconds, and if they do not break the attack, proceed with medical therapy.

The immediate goal of medical therapy is to lower the IOP. First, you should administer topical agents that decrease aqueous production, including a β-blocker, a carbonic anhydrase inhibitor, and an α-agonist. You can also give oral or intravenous acetazolamide and/or osmotic agents, such as oral isosorbide or intravenous mannitol. You should also initiate topical corticosteroid therapy (one drop every 20 minutes) to reduce the inflammation associated with the attack. If the affected eye is phakic, give pilocarpine 1% or 2% to help constrict the pupil and break the pupillary block. Miotic therapy is frequently not effective until the IOP has been reduced because of pressure-induced ischemia of the iris and paralysis of the sphincter muscle. Therefore, administration of pilocarpine should follow administration of the aqueous production inhibitors. For aphakic or pseudophakic eyes, pupil-dilating drops should be given instead.

If medical therapy is not successful in breaking an attack of acute angle closure glaucoma after 1 hour, you should consider several additional treatment options. Laser iridotomy is the definitive treatment to break the attack and reduce the risk of additional attacks. Nd:YAG laser iridotomy is often successful in breaking an attack, especially in eyes with light-colored irises. However, perforating an edematous, inflamed, thick brown iris may be difficult. Thus, for these cases, my preference is to first perform laser peripheral iridoplasty with an argon or diode laser.[2] The goal is to pull the peripheral iris away from the trabecular meshwork and allow aqueous to pass through. Using a large spot size (500 to 1000 μm), long duration (0.5 to 1 second), and low energy (100 to 250 mW), you should apply the laser spots to the far periphery with an iridotomy lens. Adjust the laser power to give a noticeable shrinkage of the iris tissue. About one spot per clock hour is sufficient, and in most cases, the attack will usually break after a few shots. You will notice a deepening of the peripheral anterior chamber, and the patient will notice prompt relief of the pain. It is worthwhile to complete the 12 iridoplasty spots to reduce the chance of a recurrent attack prior to definitive iridotomy treatment. Unlike laser iridotomy, peripheral iridoplasty works well with iris edema and even moderate corneal edema. Laser peripheral iridoplasty can also be performed as first-line treatment, prior to starting medical therapy, for rapid relief of an acute attack.[3] As an alternative to peripheral iridoplasty, a pupilloplasty can also break the pupillary block by pulling the iris pupil margin away from the anterior lens surface. Again, you are trying to achieve visible shrinking of iris tissue. Pupilloplasty may leave a noticeable distortion of the pupil afterward. However, the pupil may remain irregular after an acute angle closure attack itself due to ischemic damage to the iris sphincter.

Some clinicians advocate performing an anterior chamber paracentesis to break an acute angle closure glaucoma attack.[4] The resultant IOP drop may be sufficient to allow the pupil to react to the pilocarpine and thus break the pupillary block. If necessary, you can use a blunt cannula to push the peripheral iris posteriorly to open up the adjacent angle and relieve the attack. In my opinion, a paracentesis carries a higher risk of complication than a laser peripheral iridoplasty or pupilloplasty.

If the attack breaks with medical therapy, iridoplasty, pupilloplasty, or paracentesis, the patient will need to have definitive treatment to prevent further acute attacks and to reduce the risk of long-term IOP elevation. A laser iridotomy in both eyes is the most common treatment, but phacoemulsification may be a viable alternative.[5] Optimally, however, you should defer laser iridotomy or phacoemulsification in the involved eye until the cornea is clearer and the intraocular inflammation has improved, typically in 1 or 2 days, but occasionally longer (Figure 27-1). During and immediately after an acute attack, the iris is edematous and inflamed, such that achieving a successful laser iridotomy is more difficult. After breaking the initial attack, you should send the patient

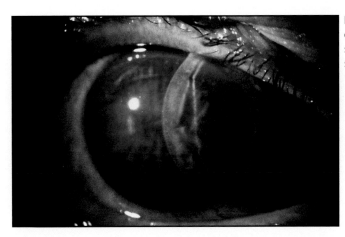

Figure 27-1. Persistent corneal edema 3 days after acute angle closure attack. (Reprinted with permission from Dale K. Heuer, MD.)

home on topical medications, including β-blocker, carbonic anhydrase inhibitor, α_2 agonist, pilocarpine (unless phacoemulsification is imminent), and corticosteroid. Emphasize to the patient that definitive treatment is still needed to prevent another attack in either eye.

In rare instances, an acute angle closure attack cannot be broken with the methods previously described. You should then perform a definitive incisional peripheral iridectomy emergently in an operating room. Do remember that the IOP often remains elevated after an angle closure attack, so plan your surgical iridectomy with the possibility that further glaucoma surgery may be needed in the future. Thus, you should use a clear corneal approach for the surgical iridectomy so the superior conjunctiva is not compromised.

As an alternative to incisional peripheral iridectomy, phacoemulsification with intraocular lens (IOL) implantation, with or without goniosynechialysis, has also been advocated in recalcitrant cases of acute angle closure glaucoma.[6] The pupillary block is relieved intraoperatively and the chamber angle widened with replacement of the natural lens with a thinner IOL implant.

If a surgical intervention is performed, remember to do a laser iridotomy in the contralateral eye if it is at risk for angle closure.

Topiramate-induced acute angle closure is caused by forward displacement of the lens-iris diaphragm by ciliochoroidal effusions as an idiosyncratic response to the medication. Immediate treatment should consist of topical aqueous suppressants, including β-blocker, α-agonist, and carbonic anhydrase inhibitors. Unlike pupillary block, miotics such as pilocarpine should be avoided. Instead, cycloplegics should be used to move the lens-iris diaphragm posteriorly. Oral carbonic anhydrase inhibitors may also cause idiosyncratic ciliochoroidal effusions and should be avoided. Topical corticosteroids can be used to control inflammation, and, of course, the inciting medication should be stopped. For recalcitrant cases, intravenous mannitol and/or methylprednisolone has been advocated,[7] but laser iridotomy would not be helpful. The condition typically resolves after a few days or weeks after cessation of topiramate.

References

1. Saw SM, Gazzard G, Friedman DS. Interventions for angle-closure glaucoma: an evidence-based update. *Ophthalmology.* 2003;110:1869-1878.
2. Lam DSC, Lai JSM, Tham CCY, Chua JKH, Poon ASY. Argon laser peripheral iridoplasty versus conventional systemic medical therapy in treatment of acute primary angle-closure glaucoma: a prospective, randomized, controlled trial. *Ophthalmology.* 2002;109:1591-1596.

3. Ritch R, Tham CC, Lam DS. Argon laser peripheral iridoplasty (ALPI): an update. *Surv Ophthalmol.* 2007;52:279-288.
4. Lam DS, Chua JK, Tham CC, Lai JS. Efficacy and safety of immediate anterior chamber paracentesis in the treatment of acute primary angle-closure glaucoma: a pilot study. *Ophthalmology.* 2002;109:64-70.
5. Husain R, Gazzard G, Aung T, et al. Initial management of acute primary angle closure: a randomized trial comparing phacoemulsification with laser peripheral iridotomy. *Ophthalmology.* 2012;119:2274-2281.
6. Harasymowycz PJ, Papamatheakis DG, Ahmed I, et al. Phacoemulsification and goniosynechialysis in the management of unresponsive primary angle closure. *J Glaucoma.* 2005;14:186-189.
7. Rhee DJ, Ramos-Esteban JC, Nipper KS. Rapid resolution of topiramate-induced angle-closure glaucoma with methylprednisolone and mannitol. *Am J Ophthalmol.* 2006;141:1133-1134.

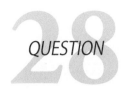

QUESTION

HOW SHOULD I MANAGE
NEOVASCULAR GLAUCOMA?

Hylton R. Mayer, MD and
James C. Tsai, MD, MBA

Neovascular glaucoma (NVG) describes a spectrum of elevated intraocular pressure (IOP) and anticipated or realized optic nerve damage caused by fibrovascular proliferation within the anterior segment of the eye (Figure 28-1). Identification of the origin of angiogenesis and appropriate intervention to reduce angiogenesis while managing IOP can prevent blinding consequences.

The physiologic mechanisms that control angiogenesis are numerous and complex. Diffusible mediators, primarily released by the retina, such as vascular endothelial growth factor (VEGF), circulate throughout the eye and promote fibrovascular proliferation. Anterior chamber neovascularization can progress through a series of clinicopathologic stages. The preglaucoma stage is characterized by the presence of anterior chamber neovascularization but normal IOP (Figure 28-2). The open-angle stage occurs when a fine fibrovascular membrane obstructs aqueous outflow, raising IOP, despite a gonioscopically open angle. The angle closure stage is the result of contraction of the fibrovascular membrane and various degrees of peripheral anterior synechiae (PAS) causing elevated IOP.[1]

Ocular ischemia is the most common inciting factor in NVG, with proliferative diabetic retinopathy, central retinal vein occlusion, and ocular ischemic syndrome accounting for the majority of cases. The underlying cause for NVG is frequently obvious, but occasionally the etiology is uncertain and requires ancillary testing and subspecialty evaluation. Table 28-1 provides an extensive list of ocular diseases in which NVG has been observed.[2]

The management of NVG requires a multifaceted approach to decrease the production of vasoproliferative factors, minimize the effect of the growth factors that are present, and control the extent of ocular hypertension (OHT) (Figure 28-3). If the retina is the source of vasoproliferative factors, as is often the case, prompt panretinal photocoagulation (PRP), usually aiming for 1500 to 2000 or more spots divided over 2 sessions, is a critical first step in controlling angiogenesis. We

Gedde SJ, ed. *Curbside Consultation in Glaucoma:*
49 Clinical Questions, Second Edition (pp 127–132)

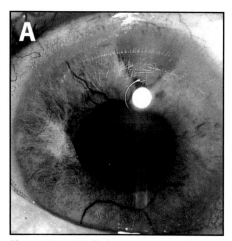 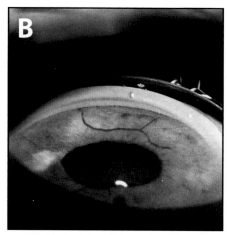

Figure 28-1. (A) Slit-lamp photograph revealing dramatic iris rubeosis. (B) Direct gonioscopy demonstrating diffuse angle closure in the presence of iris neovascularization. (Reprinted with permission from Max Forbes, MD.)

Figure 28-2. Indirect gonioscopy identifying an anterior chamber angle open to the ciliary body band with neovascularization of the iris crossing the scleral spur and arborizing in the trabecular meshwork. (Reprinted with permission from Dale K. Heuer, MD.)

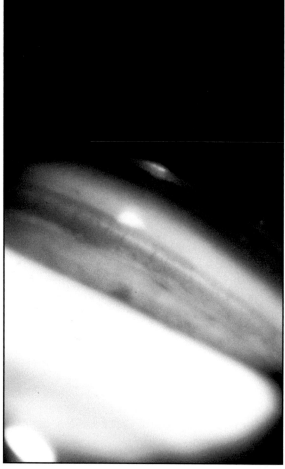

Table 28-1
Diseases Associated With Neovascular Glaucoma

Retinal Ischemic Diseases	Surgically Induced (continued)
Diabetes	Scleral buckle
Central retinal vein occlusion	Neodymium: yttrium-aluminum-garnet capsulotomy
Ocular ischemic syndrome/carotid occlusive disease	Laser coreoplasty
Central retinal artery occlusion	Tumors
Retinal detachment	Iris: melanoma, hemangioma, metastatic lesion
Leber's congenital amaurosis	Ciliary body: ring melanoma
Coats' disease	Retina: retinoblastoma, large cell lymphoma
Eales' disease	Choroid: melanoma
Sickle-cell retinopathy	Conjunctiva: squamous cell carcinoma
Retinal hemangioma	Radiation
Persistent hyperplastic primary vitreous	External beam
Norrie's disease	Charged particle: proton, helium
Wyburn-Mason's syndrome	Plaques
Carotid-cavernous fistula	Photoradiation
Dural shunt	*Inflammatory Diseases*
Stickler's syndrome	Uveitis: chronic iridocyclitis, Behçet's disease
X-linked retinoschisis	Vogt-Koyanagi-Harada syndrome
Takayasu's arteritis	Syphilitic retinitis
Juxtafoveal telangiectasia	Sympathetic ophthalmia
Surgically Induced	Endophthalmitis
Carotid endarterectomy	Miscellaneous
Cataract extraction	Vitreous wick syndrome
Pars plana vitrectomy/lensectomy	Interferon-α
Silicone oil	

Reprinted from *Ophthalmology*, 108, Sivak-Callcott JA, O'Day DM, Gass JDM, Tsai JC, Evidence-based recommendations for the diagnosis and treatment of neovascular glaucoma, 1767–1778, © 2001, with permission from Elsevier.

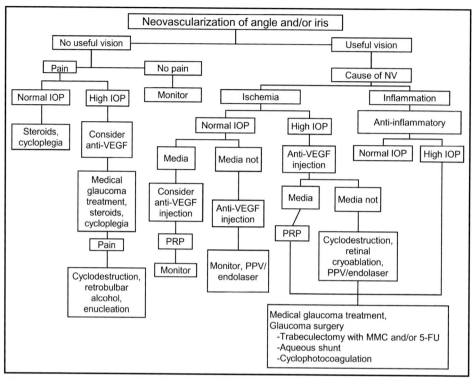

Figure 28-3. Algorithm for the management of NVG caused by ischemia and inflammation. (Adapted from an algorithm in Sivak-Callcott JA, O'Day DM, Gass JDM, Tsai JC. Evidence-based recommendations for the diagnosis and treatment of NVG. *Ophthalmology*. 2001;108:1767-1778.)

also prefer early anti-VEGF pharmacotherapy, either bevacizumab (Avastin [Genentech, San Francisco, California]) or ranibizumab (Lucentis [Genentech]). In the preglaucoma and open-angle stages of NVG (see Figure 28-2), anti-VEGF therapy can rapidly diminish the amount of neovascularization on anterior chamber structures and can occasionally obviate the need for chronic IOP-lowering therapy or surgical intervention. Preoperative anti-VEGF therapy in combination with PRP has been shown to improve surgical successes and decrease perioperative hyphema.[3] When medical IOP-lowering agents achieve reasonable IOP control, we prefer to delay surgical intervention by 3 to 7 days after injection of anti-VEGF medication to allow for adequate regression of the neovascularization. The acceptable level of IOP control varies from patient to patient, but in most instances, a patient without prior glaucomatous optic neuropathy may tolerate several days of IOP levels in the 40-mm Hg range without untoward effect. However, patients who already have glaucomatous damage or a history of retinal venous occlusion may require earlier surgical intervention.

As with most glaucomatous conditions, topical medical therapy is the preferred initial treatment for NVG. We often increase the number and intensity of topical IOP-lowering medications because of the recalcitrant nature of IOP control in patients with NVG. If there are no contraindications to a specific drug class (allergies, respiratory disease, bradycardia, etc), we often use a topical β-blocker and/or carbonic anhydrase inhibitor (CAI, including fixed combination timolol-dorzolamide), as well as an α-agonist (such as brimonidine). It is our experience that many patients will respond to prostaglandin analogues, despite the possible limited access to uveoscleral outflow pathways in advanced NVG angle closure and the coexistence of ocular inflammation. At the very least, the use of prostaglandin analogues does not seem to harm patients, even if the medications have a limited IOP-lowering effect. We prefer to avoid the use of miotic agents in NVG. We typically reserve oral carbonic anhydrase therapy for patients who have uncontrolled IOP levels despite maximum tolerated topical therapy. Although one might expect that an oral CAI agent theoretically would have little or no additional effect on aqueous production in the presence of a topical CAI, we have noted that some patients get a reasonable IOP response with the addition of a systemic CAI. In our experience, some cases of NVG that are diagnosed early and treated aggressively may develop complete regression of neovascularization, preservation of normal angle structures, and maintenance of acceptable IOP levels with few or no IOP-lowering medications. However, most of our patients with NVG present with extensive and irreversible anterior chamber structural damage for which surgical intervention is ultimately performed.

If topical or systemic IOP-lowering medications do not control IOP adequately and there is functionally useful visual potential—count fingers or better—we pursue surgical intervention. One might consider the use of primary trabeculectomy with antifibrosis therapy to obtain immediate IOP control, but numerous studies have reported an unacceptably high long-term surgical failure rate. Nevertheless, it is our opinion that trabeculectomy with mitomycin C is a reasonable surgical alternative to the use of valved and nonvalved aqueous shunts, especially when the neovascularization has regressed. Since meta-analyses have demonstrated that valved and nonvalved aqueous shunts have similar long-term outcomes, it is our opinion that either option is reasonable and acceptable and should be tailored to surgeon preference.[4]

In most cases of NVG with uncontrolled IOP levels, we prefer to use the flexible plate Ahmed drainage valve (FP7) for its ease of insertion, immediate IOP control, and lower incidence of postoperative hypotony. Our surgical procedure includes entering the anterior chamber with a 23-gauge needle and using a small amount of viscoelastic intraoperatively to help prevent significant pressure shifts intraoperatively, anterior chamber flattening, and early postoperative hypotony. If at all possible, we place the implant in the superotemporal quadrant, followed in preference by the inferotemporal or inferonasal quadrant and then by the superonasal quadrant. We use a 5 × 8-mm scleral reinforcement graft on all cases to cover the course of the tube to limit the risk of late tube erosion and exposure. We prefer to maintain topical corticosteroid therapy for approximately 3 months after drainage tube placement, tapering from 4 times a day in the first few weeks to once a day after about 2 months. During the hypertensive phase of the drainage implant, we consider adding topical IOP-lowering agents. If IOP remains elevated and/or bleb encapsulation persists, we administer a course of 3 to 5 subconjunctival 5-fluorouracil injections over the implant.

We do not believe that a role for laser peripheral iridoplasty, laser gonioplasty, or laser trabeculoplasty exists. A laser peripheral iridotomy will not improve the configuration of the angle structures in the setting of synechial closure. Most of the minimally invasive glaucoma surgeries (MIGS), such as Trabectome or iStent, are contraindicated due to the typically poor anterior chamber angle anatomy in NVG. In some circumstances, endocyclophotocoagulation (ECP) may be beneficial, especially when combined with pars plana vitrectomy (PPV), enabling more extensive treatment of the ciliary body.

If the visual potential is hand motions or worse or the patient has significant medical or social contraindications to incisional surgical intervention, we may opt to perform transscleral cyclophotocoagulation. We will perform the laser under peribulbar or retrobulbar anesthesia in the office or the operating suite. We identify the ciliary body using a Finnoff muscle light to transilluminate the globe. We usually start with 2000 mW for 2000 ms and increase the power until we hear a popping sound, indicating ciliary body eruption. Once a popping sound is identified, we decrease the power by 200 mW. We typically place 24 spots over 12 clock hours. A sub-Tenon injection of Kenalog at the end of the case may be of benefit as these patients are prone to significant postoperative inflammation. Transscleral cyclophotocoagulation may be a useful option to moderate the IOP in recalcitrant cases of NVG, while allowing time for the beneficial effects of the antiproliferative therapy (eg, PRP, anti-VEGF) to ensue and/or prepare for more definitive surgical intervention (eg, trabeculectomy with antifibrotics, aqueous shunt).

References

1. Allingham RR, Damji KF, Shields MB, et al. *Shields' Textbook of Glaucoma.* 5th ed. Philadelphia, PA: Lippincott, Williams & Wilkins; 2004.
2. Sivak-Callcott JA, O'Day DM, Gass JDM, Tsai JC. Evidence-based recommendations for the diagnosis and treatment of neovascular glaucoma. *Ophthalmology.* 2001;108:1767-1778.
3. Mahdy RA, Nada WM, Fawzy KM, et al. Efficacy of intravitreal bevacizumab with panretinal photocoagulation followed by ahmed valve implantation in neovascular glaucoma. *J Glaucoma.* 2013;22(9):768-772.
4. Minckler DS, Vedula SS, Li TJ, Mathew MC, Ayyala RS, Francis BA. Aqueous shunts for glaucoma. *Cochrane Database Syst Rev.* 2006;(2):CD004918.

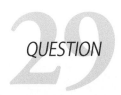
HOW SHOULD I TREAT ELEVATED INTRAOCULAR PRESSURE (WITH OR WITHOUT GLAUCOMA DAMAGE) ASSOCIATED WITH UVEITIS?

David L. Cute, DO and
Francisco Fantes, MD

The goal of management in patients with elevated intraocular pressure (IOP) associated with uveitis is to identify and treat both the underlying cause of the inflammation and the underlying mechanism(s) responsible for the IOP elevation. Determining the exact etiology of the inflammation and the mechanism(s) for the IOP elevation is vital in developing an effective, individualized treatment plan aimed at restoring a safe IOP level for the patient.

Elevated IOP in a patient with uveitis can result from an increased resistance to aqueous outflow through both open-angle and closed-angle pathogenic mechanisms, and both mechanisms may be present in some cases. When the angle is open, elevated IOP usually acutely results from decreased trabecular outflow facility caused by the accumulation of protein and inflammatory cells in the trabecular meshwork.[1] It can also result from a direct trabeculitis in cases of herpetic eye disease. In the short to intermediate term, an IOP rise can also result from corticosteroids used to control the inflammation (Figure 29-1). In the intermediate to long term, elevated IOP may stem from permanent, structural damage to the trabecular meshwork resulting from recurrent and/or prolonged inflammatory insults.

When the angle is closed, IOP elevation is most commonly caused by the organization of inflammatory debris in the angle, leading to peripheral anterior synechiae (PAS) formation. These inflammatory PAS are usually first noted in the inferior angle. Seclusion of the pupil by posterior synechiae causing iris bombé, an inflammatory ciliochoroidal effusion producing forward displacement of the lens-iris diaphragm, and inflammation-induced ischemia causing neovascularization of the angle with associated PAS formation are other, less frequent causes of secondary angle-closure associated with uveitis (Figure 29-2).[2] A thorough examination that includes dynamic gonioscopy is essential in helping to ascertain the likely mechanism behind the IOP elevation. Ancillary studies such as ultrasound biomicroscopy and B-scan ultrasonography may prove helpful in certain cases as well.

Gedde SJ, ed. *Curbside Consultation in Glaucoma:*
49 Clinical Questions, Second Edition (pp 133–140)
© 2015 Taylor & Francis Group

Figure 29-1. Slit-lamp view of sub-Tenon's depot of corticosteroid. Periocular corticosteroid injections may be helpful in controlling inflammation when frequent topical administration of corticosteroid has been inadequate but potential risk of corticosteroid-induced IOP elevation must be considered. The corticosteroid depot may need to be excised if causing unmanageable IOP elevation.

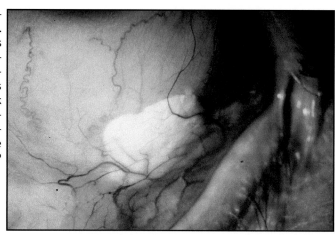

Figure 29-2. (A) Slit-lamp view of extensive posterior synechiae in a case of iridocyclitis. (B) Posterior synechiae causing pupil seclusion with iris bombé leading to subsequent closure of anterior chamber angle and increased IOP.

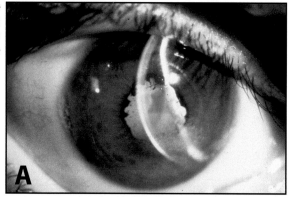

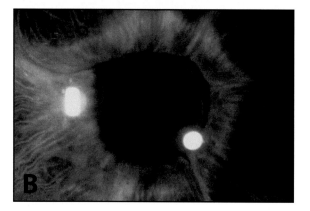

The goal of therapy is to control the inflammation and lower the IOP to a level that is thought to be safe for the patient. Medications, laser surgery, and/or incisional surgery may all be required, depending on the given scenario. When the angle is open, corticosteroids to suppress the inflammation alone may lead to adequate IOP reduction in cases of inflammation-induced, open-angle trabecular dysfunction.[1] If the use of corticosteroids alone does not promptly lower the IOP sufficiently, aqueous suppression with a topical β-blocker, α_2-agonist, and/or a carbonic anhydrase inhibitor is indicated. An oral carbonic anhydrase inhibitor can be used when adequate IOP control

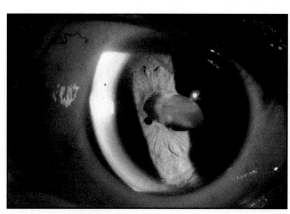

Figure 29-3. Slit-lamp view of partial lysis of posterior synechiae after administration of topical cycloplegic agents in case of chronic anterior uveitis. Cycloplegic agents may prevent or limit extent of posterior synechiae formation, thus averting progression to iris bombé and subsequent angle closure.

is not achieved with topical aqueous suppressants, and hyperosmotic agents should be considered for acute IOP elevation when urgent reduction is needed.[3] The early use of mydriatic-cycloplegic agents is helpful in preventing or breaking posterior synechiae, thus averting the possible development of a secluded pupil with iris bombé, and in stabilizing the blood-aqueous barrier (Figure 29-3). Although several controlled clinical trials have failed to show a causal relationship, the prostaglandin analogues should be used with caution in patients with uveitis due to anecdotal reports of cystoid macular edema and iridocyclitis associated with their use.[2] Miotic agents and laser trabeculoplasty are generally not effective in this setting and may possibly exacerbate the inflammation.[2,4] Keep in mind that the corticosteroid dose should be tapered to that amount necessary to control the inflammation in order to minimize any corticosteroid-induced IOP rise. Switching the topical corticosteroid agent in use to one that might have less propensity to increase the IOP while still controlling the inflammation can also be considered.[5,6] If an intravitreal corticosteroid implant is being considered, the dexamethasone implant (Ozurdex, Allergan, Inc., Irvine, CA [intravitreal implant delivered via injection through the pars plana]) has been shown to have less incidence of significant IOP rise compared with the fluocinolone acetonide implant (Retisert, Bausch & Lomb, Inc., Bridgewater, NJ [intravitreal implant delivered via pars plana incision]).[7] Corticosteroid-sparing agents can also be considered, usually requiring comanagement with a uveitis specialist. In these open-angle cases, when the maximum tolerable IOP-lowering medical therapy coupled with the minimum corticosteroid therapy needed to address the inflammation fails to achieve a safe IOP level for the patient, surgical means of achieving IOP control are indicated (Table 29-1).

Management of elevated IOP with a closed angle depends on the underlying mechanism (Table 29-2). For cases of pupillary block due to pupillary seclusion from extensive posterior synechiae or an inflammatory membrane, a laser peripheral iridotomy (LPI) is promptly indicated. Since an LPI is more prone to closure in the presence of active inflammation, it may be best to create more than one iridotomy at the time of the procedure.[1] If an LPI is not possible or repeatedly closes, an incisional peripheral iridectomy should be performed.[1,2,8] Regardless of the method used, the patient should be treated aggressively with corticosteroids both before and after the procedure to decrease the likelihood of a postoperative inflammatory flare. If an anterior shift of the lens-iris diaphragm due to ciliochoroidal effusion is the cause of the angle closure, cycloplegic agents to induce a posterior shift of the diaphragm should be used. For cases in which the angle is closed due to extensive PAS formation, with inadequately controlled IOP despite maximum tolerable medical therapy, surgical means of achieving IOP control should be considered.

Regardless of which surgical procedure is performed, an aggressive attempt to control the inflammation should be instituted preoperatively. The less preoperative inflammation, the better.

Table 29-1
Mechanisms and Management of Open-Angle Intraocular Pressure Elevation in Uveitic Patients

Mechanism of IOP Elevation	*Management*
Inflammation	Corticosteroids, aqueous suppressants, incisional surgery
Corticosteroid induced	Taper corticosteroid dose to minimum necessary, aqueous suppressants, switch to corticosteroid agent with less propensity to raise IOP, add corticosteroid-sparing agent, incisional surgery

Abbreviation: IOP, intraocular pressure.

Table 29-2
Mechanisms and Management of Closed-Angle Intraocular Pressure Elevation in Uveitic Patients

Mechanism of IOP Elevation	*Management*
Pupillary block	LPI (occasionally incisional iridectomy), aqueous suppressants
Peripheral anterior synechiae	Aqueous suppressants, incisional surgery
Ciliochoroidal effusion	Cycloplegic agents, corticosteroids

Abbreviations: IOP, intraocular pressure; LPI, laser peripheral iridotomy.

Whenever possible, surgery should be deferred until the eye has been quiescent for at least 90 days.[1] When this is not possible, especially in patients without significant optic nerve damage and in whom the IOP is not unacceptably high, it may be best to closely monitor the elevated IOP for a few weeks to allow time to gain better control of the inflammation prior to operating. When surgery cannot wait due to unacceptable IOP elevation in the presence of active inflammation, an aggressive preoperative and postoperative anti-inflammatory regimen should be instituted to minimize the surgical exacerbation of the preexisting inflammation. In all cases, so long as a significant corticosteroid-induced IOP response is not present, the preoperative corticosteroid regimen should be increased 1 week prior to the planned procedure.[1] Intraoperatively, intravenous

Table 29-3
Risks and Benefits of Different Incisional Procedures to Lower Intraocular Pressure in Uveitic Patients

Procedure	Benefits	Risks
Trabeculectomy	• Titrate IOP with suture lysis (or release) • No potential for tube-iris chafe	• Hypotony • Increased wound healing with bleb failure • Future intraocular surgery causing bleb failure
Nonvalved GDI	• Better long-term IOP reduction (compared with valved GDI) • Low risk of future intraocular surgery causing failure	• Hypotony • Tube-iris chafe increasing inflammation
Valved GDI	• Less risk of hypotony (compared with nonvalved GDI) • Low risk of future intraocular surgery causing failure	• Increased need for additional glaucoma medication for adequate IOP control • Tube-iris chafe increasing inflammation

Abbreviations: GDI, glaucoma drainage implant; IOP, intraocular pressure.

Solumedrol ([Methylprednisolone], Pfizer, Inc., NY) and/or subconjunctival dexamethasone can be used and sub-Tenon or intravitreal corticosteroids administered if the degree of inflammation warrants. Postoperatively, aggressive anti-inflammatory therapy should be maintained, and this may require the use of topical, periocular, intravitreal, and/or systemic corticosteroids.[1]

The most appropriate incisional surgery depends on the individual characteristics of each patient (Table 29-3). There are many factors to consider, including age and life expectancy of the patient, extent of glaucomatous damage, degree of active inflammation, conjunctival and scleral health, prior ophthalmic surgical history, anticoagulation status, angle configuration, and lens status. Reasonable success rates for both trabeculectomy with adjunctive antimetabolite use and glaucoma drainage implants (GDIs) in the treatment of uveitic glaucoma have been reported in the literature.[9–13] Regardless of the procedure used, we must guard against postoperative overfiltration in these eyes, many of which are already at greater risk for postoperative hypotony due to the reduced aqueous production often associated with ocular inflammatory disease.

Trabeculectomy has traditionally been the surgical procedure of choice for managing medically uncontrolled IOP in patients with uveitis.[2] In general, trabeculectomy tends to be less successful in uveitic eyes compared with nonuveitic eyes, especially if active inflammation is present at the time of surgery.[9] Even if the eye is quiet at the time of surgery, recurrent bouts of inflammation are likely to promote increased fibrous tissue growth, resulting in a decrease or loss of aqueous filtration with time. Having said that, if the conjunctiva is healthy, the inflammation is controlled, and there are no other conditions present that would significantly predispose to failure, a trabeculectomy is a reasonable first option. If trabeculectomy is chosen, an adjunctive antifibrotic agent should be used to help counter the exuberant wound-healing response often seen in uveitic patients that increases the risk of bleb failure. However, to protect against overfiltration and the risk of hypotony, tight flap closure is advised. Postoperative flap suture lysis (or release of releasable sutures) can be performed as necessary to titrate the IOP to an acceptable level.

GDIs offer an alternative surgical approach to trabeculectomy and are a popular choice in managing medically uncontrolled glaucoma in patients with ocular inflammation.[10-13] These devices are more likely to control IOP than trabeculectomy when active inflammation is present at the time of surgery and/or is very likely to be significant following surgery.[9,12] In addition, GDIs are more likely than trabeculectomy to be less adversely affected and maintain IOP control should future nonglaucoma-related ocular incisional procedures, such as phacoemulsification, be needed, which often is the case in patients with ocular inflammatory disease.[13]

Among the more commonly used GDIs today, favorable results have been reported with both the Baerveldt (nonvalved) (Abbott Medical Optics, Abbott Park, IL) and Ahmed (valved) (New World Medical, Inc., Rancho Cucamonga, CA) GDIs in eyes with uveitic glaucoma.[10,11,13] In patients with high-risk glaucoma, the Baerveldt-350 has been reported to be more effective in reducing IOP and the need for IOP-reducing medications than the Ahmed-FP7, but it also is associated with more hypotony-related complications.[14] Each device has its advantages and disadvantages in the setting of uveitic glaucoma, and the best device to use depends on the individual case. A valved device would be the better option in those patients requiring prompt, reliable IOP reduction or who are believed to be, in the surgeon's best judgment, at greater risk of developing significant, postoperative hypotony. When the preoperative IOP is not excessively high and prompt IOP reduction is not needed, so long as the risk of postoperative hypotony is not excessive, the larger Baerveldt-350 or Baerveldt-250 implant is likely the better choice as it has been associated with less bleb encapsulation, resulting in better IOP control with less need for glaucoma medications over the long term than the Ahmed-FP7.[14] One must remember that there can be increased inflammation after ligature release in patients with a nonvalved implant, and the patient's postoperative corticosteroid regimen should be adjusted to account for this.

It is also worth mentioning that significant inflammation following either routine or complicated cataract surgery can lead to marked IOP elevation in both uveitic and nonuveitic eyes. In this setting, inflammation, such as that which may be associated with retained lens material, toxic anterior segment syndrome (TASS), and uveitis-glaucoma-hyphema (UGH) syndrome, can lead to elevation of the IOP in an open-angle configuration. UGH syndrome usually results from poorly fitting anterior chamber intraocular lenses (AC IOLs), iris-supported IOLs, and ciliary sulcus placement of one-piece posterior chamber intraocular lenses (PC IOLs), which are intended only for endocapsular fixation. The optics and/or haptics of a malpositioned or unstable IOL incite chronic inflammation as well as pigment dispersion and intermittent bleeding from iris or ciliary body chafing that can overwhelm the trabecular meshwork. TASS is a profound noninfectious inflammation seen in the immediate postoperative setting resulting from problems with any solutions injected intracamerally during the procedure or problems related to the cleaning and sterilization of the instruments used during the procedure.[15] Permanent damage to the trabecular meshwork may ensue. Retained lens material following cataract surgery can also incite significant intraocular inflammation that can cause IOP elevation.

For IOP elevation in cases of UGH syndrome (Figure 29-4), topical corticosteroids and aqueous suppressants will often help to suppress the inflammation and control the IOP. Miotic or cycloplegic agents can be prescribed to limit iris movement against the IOL in an attempt to reduce or eliminate any associated iritis, pigment dispersion, or bleeding. For those cases not responding adequately to medical therapy, removal or exchange of the IOL, with its potential associated intraoperative risks, should be considered and may constitute definitive management. Cases of ocular

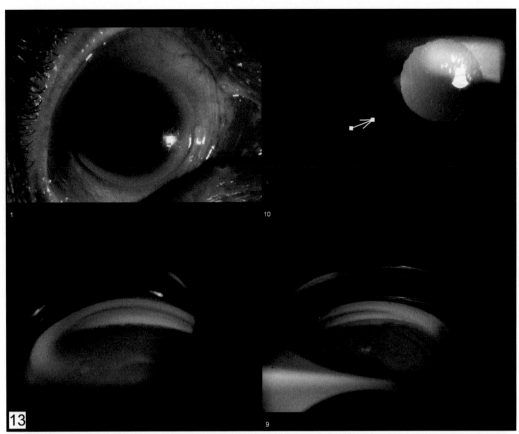

Figure 29-4. UGH syndrome, right eye, resulting from ciliary sulcus placement of one-piece PC-IOL. Upper right: inferotemporal iris transillumination defects caused by iris chafing of IOL. Bottom: gonioscopic image of relatively heavy pigmentation of trabecular meshwork due to iris pigment dispersion from iris chafing in the affected eye (left photo) compared with the uninvolved eye (right photo).

hypertension associated with TASS are best managed with aggressive anti-inflammatory therapy initially; however, topical aqueous suppressants may also be needed. IOP elevation resulting from retained lens material after cataract surgery should be managed with aggressive topical corticosteroids and aqueous suppressants, but removal of the retained lens fragments, especially if nuclear, via an anterior or posterior approach depending on the given situation, may be required to control both the inflammation and IOP. Keep in mind that permanent damage to the trabecular meshwork may ensue from any case of severe postoperative inflammation, which may necessitate long-term IOP-lowering medical therapy and/or incisional glaucoma surgery.[16]

The views expressed in this article are those of the authors and do not necessarily reflect the official policy or position of the Department of the Navy, Department of the Army, Department of Defense, or United States Government.

Acknowledgments

This chapter is dedicated to the memory of Francisco Fantes, MD, a consummate physician, mentor, and friend.

References

1. Buggage R. Uveitic Glaucomas. In: Rhee DJ, ed. *Glaucoma: Color Atlas & Synopsis of Clinical Ophthalmology.* New York, NY: McGraw-Hill; 2003:254-285.
2. Kuchtey RW, Lowder CY, Smith SD. Glaucoma in patients with ocular inflammatory disease. *Ophthalmol Clin North Am.* 2005;18:421-430.
3. Allingham RR, Damji KF, Freedman S, Moroi SE, Shafranov G. *Shields' Textbook of Glaucoma.* 5th ed. Philadelphia, PA: Lippincott Williams & Wilkins; 2005.
4. Robin AL, Pollack IP. Argon laser trabeculoplasty in secondary forms of open-angle glaucoma. *Arch Ophthalmol.* 1983;101:382-384.
5. Foster CS, Alter G, DeBarge LR, et al. Efficacy and safety of rimexolone 1% ophthalmic suspension vs 1% prednisolone acetate in the treatment of uveitis. *Am J Ophthalmol.* 1996;122(2):171-182.
6. Novack GD, Howes J, Crockett RS, et al. Change in intraocular pressure during long-term use of loteprednol etabonate. *J Glaucoma.* 1998;7:266-269.
7. Arcinue CA, Cerón OM, Foster CS. A comparison between the fluocinolone acetonide (Retisert) and dexamethasone (Ozurdex) intravitreal implants in uveitis. *J Ocul Pharmacol Ther.* 2013;29(5):501-507.
8. Kok H, Barton K. Uveitic glaucoma. *Ophthalmol Clin North Am.* 2002;15:375-387.
9. Ceballos EM, Beck AD, Lynn MJ. Trabeculectomy with antiproliferative agents in uveitic glaucoma. *J Glaucoma.* 2002;11(3):189-196.
10. Da Mata A, Burk SE, Netland PA, et al. Management of uveitic glaucoma with Ahmed glaucoma valve implantation. *Ophthalmology.* 1999;106(11):2168-2172.
11. Papadaki TG, Zacharopoulos IP, Pasquale LR, et al. Long-term results of Ahmed glaucoma valve implantation for uveitic glaucoma. *Am J Ophthalmol.* 2007;144(1):62-69.
12. Hill RA, Nguyen QH, Baerveldt G, et al. Trabeculectomy and Molteno implantation for glaucomas associated with uveitis. *Ophthalmology.* 1993;100:903-908.
13. Ceballos EM, Parrish RK, Schiffman JC. Outcome of Baerveldt glaucoma drainage implants for the treatment of uveitic glaucoma. *Ophthalmology.* 2002;109:2256-2260.
14. Christakis PG, Tsai JC, Kalenak JW, et al. The Ahmed versus Baerveldt study: three-year treatment outcomes. *Ophthalmology.* 2013;120(11):2232-2240.
15. Mamalis N. Following uneventful surgery, three of my eight patients have 4+ cell and fibrin on postoperative day 1. What should I do? In: Chang DF, ed. *Curbside Consultation in Cataract Surgery: 49 Clinical Questions.* Thorofare, NJ: SLACK Incorporated; 2007:195-198.
16. Lewis RA. What is the best way to prevent and manage postoperative intraocular pressure spikes? In: Chang DF, ed. *Curbside Consultation in Cataract Surgery: 49 Clinical Questions.* Thorofare, NJ: SLACK Incorporated; 2007:187-189.

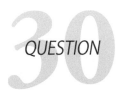

HOW SHOULD CHILDREN WITH CONGENITAL GLAUCOMA BE FOLLOWED?

Wendy W. Huang, MD

Determining appropriate follow-up for children with congenital glaucoma is complex and case dependent. When establishing a timeline for office visits and examinations under anesthesia (EUA), several factors come into play, including pathology, stability of disease, severity of disease, and patient reliability. Determining what data are necessary to make clinical decisions and when this information must be collected is key. A growing number of studies have found that early exposure to anesthesia in childhood is related to long-term cognitive development impairment. It appears this risk increases with longer cumulative exposure time to anesthesia and is also related to age at time of exposure.[1] However, one of the limitations of these studies is selection bias. Most children without issues do not undergo anesthesia at a young age and are therefore not included in the studied groups. In any case, it is important to try and avoid early, frequent EUAs as much as possible without compromising patient care.

When thinking about congenital glaucoma, pathology is the first factor I like to consider. Patients can be split into 2 main categories: glaucoma from isolated trabeculodysgenesis and glaucoma in the setting of a syndrome or other ocular anomalies, such as aniridia, Lowe syndrome, Sturge-Weber syndrome, and Axenfeld-Rieger syndrome. Patients in the latter category often have a clinical course that can be unpredictable and less responsive to angle surgery.

The next factor is the stability of the patient's disease. This can be the most challenging and difficult to assess. Stability can be defined as no abnormal growth of the eye, no anterior and posterior segment examination changes, no optic nerve changes, and no need for modification in medications to maintain normal intraocular pressure (IOP). A baseline must first be established. When an infant presents with signs characteristic of congenital glaucoma, it is important to try and arrange for an EUA within 1 to 2 weeks of presentation as long as the child is medically stable. This visit to the operating room may also include surgery on one or both eyes. As such, the person performing the EUA should be comfortable with performing surgery in this patient population

Gedde SJ, ed. *Curbside Consultation in Glaucoma:*
49 Clinical Questions, Second Edition (pp 141–143)
© 2015 Taylor & Francis Group

and have had a discussion with the parents beforehand. For a baseline, the following measures should be checked: IOP (can use Perkins Tonometer [Haag-Streit, Mason, Ohio] or Tono-Pen [Reichert Technologies, Depew, New York]), refraction, central corneal thickness, corneal diameter, and axial length. An anterior and posterior segment examination, including gonioscopy, should be performed. Optic disc photos and pertinent anterior segment photos should be obtained. If surgery is performed, I usually see the patient in the office on postoperative day 1 and week 1 to ensure that there is no infection. A follow-up EUA is then scheduled for a new postoperative baseline. If the IOP is controlled and easily obtained, the examination can be performed in the office and a repeat EUA a few months later.

The most difficult part of the in-office examination of a child is obtaining an accurate IOP. When this is not possible, a trip to the operating room is often required. With the advent of the iCare rebound tonometer (Tiolat Ot, Helsinki, Finland), the need for examinations under anesthesia has been reduced.[2] No anesthetic drops are required for rebound tonometry, resulting in IOP measurements with little irritation to the patient; however, the child must be upright. Recent studies have suggested that although IOP by rebound tonometry correlates well with Goldmann tonometry, there is a tendency to overestimate IOP, particularly in children with glaucoma.[3,4]

Severity of disease is another factor that dictates management. Patients who are functionally monocular, have failed several surgical treatments, have significant optic disc cupping in one or both eyes, have significant anisometropia, or are legally blind need frequent monitoring. Most patients in this population are within amblyopic age. They require, at minimum, 3- to 4-month interval vision checks to ensure amblyopia is properly treated. Patients with congenital glaucoma can have rapidly increasing myopia and anisometropia from asymmetric disease. As such, without proper follow-up, the severity of their disease can outpace clinical findings.

The last factor to weigh is the patient's reliability for follow-up. The pediatric population is particularly vulnerable to social issues. Children depend on adults to bring them to appointments, deliver medications, and enforce patching and glasses. Proper understanding of how well these tasks can be executed and assessing the risk of loss to follow-up is essential. It requires working with families, social workers, and child services in some cases to establish a line of communication. Often times, investing time early on to educate parents about long-term prognosis without proper care can avoid future complications and lapses in care. More frequent visits than typically indicated may be needed as a means to educate caregivers and ensure treatments are being administered as prescribed.

With all these elements taken into consideration, the following questions can be used as a guide in establishing the timing of the next in-office examination (Figure 30-1): (1) Does the child require medication for IOP control? (2) Has the child been stable? (3) Does the child have severe glaucoma? (4) Does the current examination indicate a change in treatment? Answering these questions can be difficult. Timing of visits is very case dependent, and Figure 30-1 can be used as a guide (not a rule) to help in the management of these complex cases. Each examination in the office should have a reliable IOP reading, age-appropriate vision assessment, and an anterior/posterior segment examination. If the child is cooperative with IOP checks in the office, an EUA need only be performed once every 3 to 4 months if photographs and axial length measurements cannot be obtained in the office.

As soon as the patient is cooperative, I like to perform a visual field and repeat this test at least once a year. Goldmann visual fields, if available, are often the best measure in a child. A Humphrey visual field can be performed as well, and I recommend using a size V stimulus since this helps the patient become better accustomed to the test. Often, visual fields need to be repeated due to variability in quality and to promote familiarity with the test. Results can initially vary when the child is first learning how to do the test.

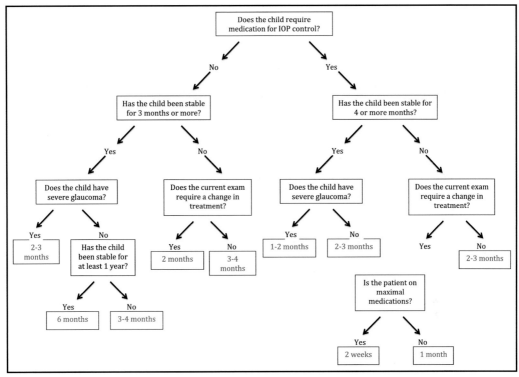

Figure 30-1. Algorithm for approximate timing of the next in-office examination.

Management of congenital glaucoma is case dependent and complex. All in all, by focusing on the patient's pathology, stability, severity, and reliability, the number of examinations requiring anesthesia can be minimized without compromising care.

References

1. Wilder RT, Flick RP, Sprung J, et al. Early exposure to anesthesia and learning disabilities in a population-based birth cohort. *Anesthesiology*. 2009;110(4):796-804.
2. Grigorian F, Grigorian AP, Olitsky SE. The use of the iCare tonometer reduced the need for anesthesia to measure intraocular pressure in children. *J AAPOS*. 2012;16(6):508-510.
3. Lambert SR, Melia M, Buffenn AN, Chiang MF, Simpson JL, Yang MB. Rebound tonometry in children: a report by the American Academy of Ophthalmology. *Ophthalmology*. 2013;120(4):e21-e27.
4. Dahlmann-Noor AH, Puertas R, Tabasa-Lim S, et al. Comparison of handheld rebound tonometry with Goldmann applanation tonometry in children with glaucoma: a cohort study. *BMJ Open*. 2013;3(4):e001788.

SECTION IV

MEDICAL THERAPY

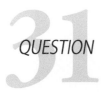

ARE ANY NEW MEDICATIONS IN DEVELOPMENT? ARE ANY NEUROPROTECTIVE AGENTS CURRENTLY AVAILABLE FOR TREATING GLAUCOMA?

Sarah R. Wellik, MD

It is now recognized that glaucoma is a neurodegenerative disease associated with long-term retinal ganglion cell death. Causes are known to be multifactorial, and although elevation of intraocular pressure (IOP) is important, other treatment strategies are being investigated. Current studies are looking toward targeting novel pathways that may protect retinal ganglion cells directly or indirectly (Figure 31-1).

New medications currently in development include Rho-kinase (ROCK) inhibitors. ROCK inhibitors were initially targeted because they lower IOP via a previously untapped pathway. The Rho family includes Rho (RhoA, RhoB, RhoC), Rac, and CDC42, which are all small G-proteins. These activate when bound to guanosine diphosphate (GDP), and the downstream effects are polymerization of actin stress fibers, forming focal adhesions. Experimental evidence indicates that the actin cytoskeleton is more disorganized in eyes with glaucoma. Therefore, ROCK inhibitors may have a positive effect on aqueous outflow, particularly in the glaucomatous trabecular meshwork. ROCK inhibitors also increase blood flow by inhibiting calcium sensitization and relaxing vascular smooth muscles. Several early human trials have shown safety and efficacy of candidate ROCK inhibitors in lowering IOP in glaucoma and ocular hypertension.[1] Reported side effects have been conjunctival hyperemia and conjunctival hemorrhage with no clinically significant effects on blood pressure or pulse rate. It has also been postulated that ROCK inhibitors have a potential for neuroprotective effects, independent of their IOP-lowering ability.[2]

A 2013 Cochrane review of neuroprotective agents for glaucoma identified only one study that met criteria for evidence as a neuroprotective agent.[3] The Low-pressure Glaucoma Treatment Study (LoGTS) was conducted to show whether brimonidine could be used as a neuroprotective agent. Although it has been shown to protect retinal ganglion cells in animal models by inhibition of the N-Methyl-D-aspartic acid (NMDA) receptor function and modulation of presynaptic glutamate release, the exact neuroprotective mechanism of brimonidine in humans is unknown. The

Gedde SJ, ed. *Curbside Consultation in Glaucoma:*
49 Clinical Questions, Second Edition (pp 147–149)
© 2015 Taylor & Francis Group

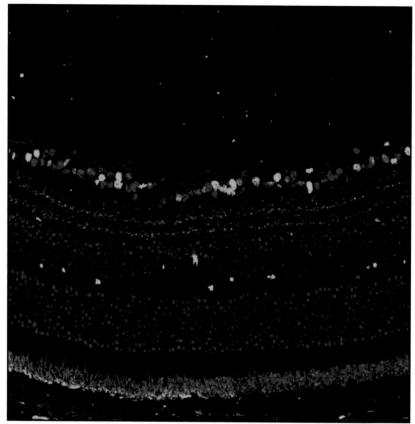

Figure 31-1. Laminated structure of the 3 retinal nuclear layers: the top layer is the retinal ganglion cell layer (RGC). Antibody linked to a green flurophore shows individual RGCs labeled in green. Orange lines are part of the inner plexiform layer and are specifically those that are derived from the RGC. (Reprinted with permission of Richard Lee, MD, PhD.)

LoGTS enrolled 190 adults and randomized them to treatment with brimonidine 0.2% or timolol 0.5%, with the primary outcome measure being visual field progression after 4 years of treatment. The major flaws of the study included a large dropout rate prior to the 4-year completion date (with a proportionately larger number of brimonidine dropouts). Bearing this in mind, fewer patients in the brimonidine group had visual field progression at the 4-year follow-up while IOP was similar in both groups (14.2 mm Hg in the brimonidine group and 14.0 mm Hg in the timolol group). The study did not report certain secondary outcome measures that may have been significant such as visual acuity and changes in the cup-to-disc ratio.

Memantine is another drug that was tested in phase III clinical trials for glaucoma, although specific data have not been released to date. Memantine (an NMDA receptor antagonist) was approved for use in Alzheimer disease, and 2 separate phase III clinical trials were done to show whether it could be used for glaucoma neuroprotection. The first trial showed that this medication slowed progression of glaucoma. However, a press release from Allergan after the second phase III trial stated that "although the study showed that the progression of disease was significantly lower in patients receiving the higher dose of memantine compared to patients receiving the low dose of memantine, there was no significant benefit compared to patients receiving placebo. Therefore, the study failed to meet its primary endpoint and to sufficiently replicate the results of the first phase III trial." This was a long and costly multicenter trial that had high expectations, but it resulted in no marketable therapy.

Other potential neuroprotective agents that have been studied include nipradilol (a β-blocker with nitric oxide donative action), oral brovincamine fumarate (a calcium channel blocker), ω-3 fatty acids, cannabinoids, ginkgo biloba (an antioxidant that may also interfere with the NMDA receptor), melatonin, and vitamin B_{12}. Although some studies published positive results, others did not, and none proved feasible to do larger human trials. Future directions include the possibility of using nanoparticles, which could be coupled with glaucoma drugs, glial cell neurotrophic factors, or to deliver gene therapy.

Neuroprotection trials are fraught with difficulty. Glaucoma is a disease with a long, slow course that is often asymptomatic. Monitoring for definitive progression can be a challenge as visual field tests can be plagued by patient variability. It will be necessary in future glaucoma clinical trials to come up with alternative testing strategies. This could include testing candidate drugs in smaller populations with a higher threshold for success and identifying patients with higher risk for rapid disease progression or "fast progressors" where a treatment effect could be elucidated in less time.[4] New strategies for drug testing may also include using Web-based technology to establish an electronic network of physicians at various academic centers and nonacademic clinical practices, as has been used in other areas of ophthalmology (Diabetic Retinopathy Clinical Research Network). This may make it possible to rapidly identify potential study patients while collectively minimizing bureaucratic requirements.

Future trends in glaucoma treatments include not only exploiting what we now know about the biochemical pathways of trabecular meshwork but also incorporating new ideas for drug delivery and testing.

References

1. Tanihara H, Inoue T, Yamamoto T, Kuwayama Y, Abe H, Arale M; K-115 Clinical Study Group. Phase 2 randomized clinical study of a Rho kinase inhibitor, K-115, in primary open-angle glaucoma and ocular hypertension. *Am J Ophthalmol.* 2013;156(4):731-736.
2. Inoue T, Tanihara H. Rho-associated kinase inhibitors: a novel glaucoma therapy. *Prog Retin Eye Res.* 2013;37:1-12.
3. Sena DF, Lindsley K. Neuroprotection for treatment of glaucoma in adults. *Cochrane Database Syst Rev.* 2013;(2):CD006539.
4. Quigley HA. Clinical trials for glaucoma neuroprotection are not impossible. *Curr Opin Ophthalmol.* 2012;23(2):144-154.

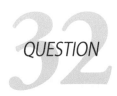

QUESTION

WHICH GLAUCOMA MEDICATIONS CAN BE SAFELY USED DURING PREGNANCY? IN CHILDHOOD?

Bhavna P. Sheth, MD, MBA

Medical treatment of glaucoma in pregnancy and childhood requires review of the risks and benefits of treatment for both the mother and the child. Information in the literature regarding the safety of glaucoma medications in pregnancy and childhood has been gathered predominantly by clinicians' experiences and case reports, as well as the review of systemic forms of the topical medications.[1]

Pregnancy

Patients with glaucoma need ongoing surveillance during pregnancy because the course of glaucoma may be variable.[2] Some patients may be successfully followed without treatment, whereas other patients may need medical or surgical treatment during pregnancy.

Intraocular pressure (IOP) has a tendency to decrease during pregnancy, which may allow certain patients to be monitored on reduced medications or without treatment during pregnancy. In addition, young patients with early glaucoma may tolerate small increases in the IOP during pregnancy without any apparent adverse effect. Furthermore, some patients may opt to be monitored off of medications because of the concern of teratogenic adverse effects. I believe this is a reasonable approach for those patients with early or mild disease in whom the risk of significant damage is small during the course of pregnancy.

When treatment is considered during pregnancy, the practitioner needs to engage the patient and her obstetrician in the decision-making process. Although there is limited information regarding the safety of glaucoma medications in pregnancy, the US Food and Drug Administration (FDA) drug classification system, as well as published reports on the use of various glaucoma agents during pregnancy, can be used for guidance. The FDA drug classification system labels

Gedde SJ, ed. *Curbside Consultation in Glaucoma: 49 Clinical Questions, Second Edition* (pp 151–153)
© 2015 Taylor & Francis Group

Table 32-1
Food and Drug Administration Pregnancy Categories

Category	Description	Medications
A	Studies in pregnant women have not shown an increased risk to the fetus	
B	Animal studies have revealed no harm to the fetus, but no studies have been done in pregnant women; or animal studies have shown an adverse effect, but studies in pregnant women have failed to demonstrate a risk to the fetus	Brimonidine and dipivefrin
C	No animal studies have been performed and it is not known whether the drug can cause harm when given to pregnant women; or animal studies have shown an adverse effect, but there are no studies in pregnant women	Timolol, betaxolol, dorzolamide/timolol, dorzolamide, brinzolamide, latanoprost, bimatoprost, travoprost, and pilocarpine
D	Drug can cause fetal harm when administered to a pregnant woman	
X	Drug is contraindicated in women who are or may become pregnant	

drugs based on information gathered by human and animal studies (Table 32-1). Most glaucoma medications are category C, indicating that either no animal studies have been performed or that animal studies have shown an adverse effect but no studies in humans are available. If topical medications are used, systemic absorption should be minimized with the use of punctal occlusion.

Dipivefrin hydrochloride and brimonidine tartrate are the only 2 category B medications. Category B medications indicate presumed safety based on animal studies. Brimonidine, an α_2 adrenergic agonist, has been reported to be used in pregnancy without adverse effect, and it tends to be one of my agents of choice (along with topical β-blockers). However, due to the possibility of respiratory and central nervous system depression in neonates, it should be avoided near the term of pregnancy.

Several other glaucoma medications have been used during pregnancy with and without adverse events. There has been significant experience with the use of systemic β-blockers for controlling blood pressure in pregnancy, and therefore this class of medication is often considered as a reasonable option for the treatment of pregnant women with glaucoma. Case reports have indicated the safe use of topical β-blockers during pregnancy, although there was one case of fetal bradycardia with the use of topical timolol by the mother. Several case reports have also indicated the safe use of topical carbonic anhydrase inhibitors (CAIs) during pregnancy. Oral administration of CAIs has been reported to have adverse effects in 2 case reports (one case of teratoma and another of electrolyte abnormalities in offspring of patients treated with oral acetazolamide). However, oral administration of acetazolamide for the treatment of idiopathic intracranial hypertension did not appear to have adverse effect on maternal or fetal outcome in a retrospective study.[3] Although there is insufficient clinical or experimental evidence to support adverse effects of oral CAIs on pregnancy outcomes, I would still use them with extreme caution in pregnancy and only after appropriate informed consent.

Prostaglandin analogues should be avoided during pregnancy since animal studies have revealed the increased risk of abortion or preterm delivery with the systemic use of this class of drugs. Interestingly, one author did report on 11 women who were exposed to latanoprost during the first trimester of pregnancy without any adverse pregnancy or neonatal outcomes.[4] While the safe use of topical pilocarpine has been reported during pregnancy, this agent may not be ideal in young patients with glaucoma due to its other side effects of induced myopia and brow ache.

Some patients may demonstrate progression of their glaucoma during pregnancy. Alternative therapies, such as laser trabeculoplasty or incisional surgery, may be employed in those patients who are at significant risk of progressive vision or visual field loss despite medical therapy. There are no published data regarding the effectiveness of laser trabeculoplasty in pregnancy. The success rate of trabeculectomy or aqueous shunts is presumably relatively similar to that in other patients of similar ages with a similar glaucoma diagnosis and ocular surgical history. However, 5-fluorouracil and mitomycin should not be used with trabeculectomy in pregnant women.

Children

Although childhood glaucoma is often treated surgically, medical treatment can be used before surgery or can supplement surgical therapy. As in pregnancy, clinicians should review the risks and benefits of medical treatment, use the lowest dose necessary, monitor for any ocular and systemic adverse effects, and provide instruction on the use of punctal occlusion.

Topical β-blockers and CAIs, as well as the fixed combination of timolol and dorzolamide, have been used in children to lower IOP. The FDA labeling of Timolol GFS 0.25% (Falcon Pharmaceuticals Ltd [division of Alcon, Fort Worth, Texas]) and 0.5% and Betoptic S 0.25% (Alcon) indicates that the safety of these drugs has been demonstrated in pediatric patients based on a 3-month multicenter trial. Topical β-blockers may be associated with apnea and bradycardia and thus should be used with caution in neonates. Treatment should be initiated with the lowest dose possible and the subsequent ocular and systemic response monitored. The topical α_2-agonist, brimonidine, has been associated with central nervous system depression, somnolence, and apnea, and thus it should be avoided in neonates and children younger than 2 years. Prostaglandin analogues, such as latanoprost, have been used in children with variable efficacy and with local side effects similar to those seen in adults.

References

1. Maris PJ Jr, Mandal AK, Netland PA. Medical therapy of pediatric glaucoma and glaucoma in pregnancy. *Ophthalmol Clin North Am.* 2005;18:461-468.
2. Brauner SC, Chen TC, Hutchinson BT, Chang MA, Pasquale LR, Grosskreutz CL. The course of glaucoma during pregnancy: a retrospective case series. *Arch Ophthalmol.* 2006;124:1089-1094.
3. Falardeau, J, Lobb BM, Golden S, Maxfield SD, Tanne E. The use of acetazolamide during pregnancy in intracranial hypertension patients. *J Neuroophthalmol.* 2013;33(1):8-12.
4. De Santis M, Lucchese A, Carducci B, et al. Latanoprost exposure in pregnancy. *Am J Ophthalmol.* 2004;138:305-306.

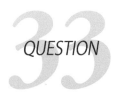

IS THERE STILL A ROLE FOR MIOTICS IN SOME PATIENTS? ORAL CARBONIC ANHYDRASE INHIBITORS?

Richard K. Lee, MD, PhD

The introduction of the prostaglandin analogues has significantly changed our prescription patterns and even the frequency of surgery for the treatment of glaucoma. Partly because of the excellent safety profile (minimal systemic side effects), ease of use (daily dosing), and efficacy of this class of topical medications, the use of other classes of glaucoma medications has decreased in frequency as the prostaglandin analogues have become the most frequently used drug class to treat glaucoma. Nonetheless, a significant role exists for the use of miotics and oral carbonic anhydrase inhibitors (CAIs) in certain glaucoma populations.

Miotics and CAIs are used to decrease intraocular pressure (IOP) through different mechanisms of action. Miotics are cholinergic agonists working either at the level of cholinergic receptors (direct acting) or by inhibiting cholinesterases (indirect acting) to increase the effective amount of acetylcholine as a cholinergic agonist. Miotics are believed to work mainly by mechanically contracting the ciliary muscle and widening the trabecular meshwork channels to increase aqueous outflow facility and by pulling the iris away from the trabecular meshwork in eyes with narrow angles to lower the IOP.[1] CAIs decrease IOP by decreasing aqueous humor production by the ciliary body.[2]

Miotics are one of the oldest classes of glaucoma medications, but as its usage has decreased with the introduction of new classes of topical medications, so has the number of commercially readily available choices for these cholinergic agents. Pilocarpine and carbachol are commercially available topical direct-acting cholinergic agonists. Pilocarpine is the most widely available topical miotic, although carbachol can be ordered through a wholesaler by a community pharmacy if it is not stocked on the pharmacy shelf. Echothiophate iodide is an indirect cholinesterase inhibitor and is only available by drop shipment through a wholesaler or ordered directly from the manufacturer. The manufacturer for echothiophate iodide will provide the medication for patients with

Gedde SJ, ed. *Curbside Consultation in Glaucoma:
49 Clinical Questions, Second Edition* (pp 155–157)
© 2015 Taylor & Francis Group

glaucoma if other glaucoma medications are not effective or for patients who have been maintained on echothiophate iodide.

The use of miotics has decreased partially because of their side effect profile compared with some of the new glaucoma medications. Cholinergic agonists can worsen vision loss associated with cataracts and dark environments because of miosis (although patients who tolerate miotics often enjoy the pinhole effect), worsen ocular inflammation (especially in association with uveitis and ocular surgery), increase the risk of retinal detachment, possibly increase scarring of the conjunctiva (which may affect future glaucoma surgery), cause atrophy of the iris pupillary dilator muscle (making dilation difficult for cataract surgery), induce myopia, and precipitate angle closure (secondary to pupillary block). Systemic side effects include those commonly associated with cholinergic stimulation such as diarrhea, decreased bladder control, abdominal cramps, brow ache (due to ciliary body spasm), cardiac function changes, and bronchial obstruction.[1] Indirect miotics in particular have a higher frequency of inducing iris pigment epithelial cysts, punctual stenosis, pseudopemphigoid, cataract formation, and depletion of cholinesterases.

Acetazolamide and methazolamide are the only oral CAIs commercially available for the treatment of glaucoma. The oral CAIs are often regarded as a last line therapy for the treatment of glaucoma because of their systemic side effects, which include electrolyte imbalances (especially hypokalemia and metabolic acidosis), urolithiasis, idiosyncratic aplastic anemia, Stevens-Johnson syndrome, and thrombocytopenia. The oral CAIs are contraindicated in patients with sulfonamide allergies and should be used cautiously in patients with renal disease. Many patients stop oral CAIs because of intolerance due to constitutional side effects such as fatigue, malaise, gastric upset, altered taste, paresthesias, and decreased appetite.[2]

Pilocarpine, the most commonly used miotic, is indicated for treatment of open-angle glaucoma (OAG) but is infrequently used now because of its side effect profile and increased frequency of dosing (QID) relative to other glaucoma medications. However, miotics are an important consideration in the effective treatment of pigmentary glaucoma (where miotics decrease pigment shedding) and plateau iris glaucoma (where miotics pull the peripheral iris away from the trabecular meshwork and widen the angle). In addition, miotics are helpful prior to laser peripheral iridotomy (LPI) in aiding peripheral placement of an iridotomy. Miotics can also help break synechiae (with alternating mydriatic use). I have tried switching some patients with moderate tolerance of pilocarpine to prostaglandin analogues and have occasionally found marked IOP elevation as a result. Thus, miotics may play a unique role in controlling IOP compared with other glaucoma medications in some patients. I use pilocarpine as a last-line therapy in patients who have failed other glaucoma medications or who require greater IOP lowering but are reluctant to undergo surgery. I typically start patients on 1% or 2% pilocarpine QID and increase the percentage (up to 4%) depending on tolerance, efficacy, and iris pigmentation (pilocarpine is bound by pigment; darker eyed patients may need higher concentrations).[1]

Oral CAIs are potent pressure-lowering medications. However, poor patient tolerance has been a barrier to more frequent use. Nonetheless, certain patients with glaucoma can be treated efficaciously with oral CAIs, especially if these patients are reluctant to have or are poor candidates for glaucoma surgery and/or have intolerance to topical glaucoma medications. Oral CAIs are also great for bilateral IOP control in patients with poor compliance (some patients are more likely to take pills than drops) or in patients who have difficulty instilling eye drops. Oral CAIs are underused, partly because of past experiences with poor acetazolamide tolerance. Acetazolamide appears to be more potent in lowering IOP but is associated with a much higher incidence of intolerance. Patients who do not tolerate acetazolamide often tolerate methazolamide well.[3] Oral CAIs act relatively quickly and potently, in conjunction with topical glaucoma medications, to lower IOP acutely and are an important adjunct to therapy for acute glaucoma, recalcitrant elevated IOP (ie, neovascular glaucoma), and routine glaucoma treatment. When using an oral CAI, I typically start patients on methazolamide (50 mg PO BID) and titrate up or down by dose (up to 100 mg) and frequency (down to QD or up to TID) depending on tolerance and side effects. Patients with renal disease or using other potassium-wasting diuretics (eg, hydrochlorothiazide, furosemide) should be monitored for electrolyte changes when oral CAIs are used. Oral and topical CAIs have similar efficacy for lowering IOP, and topical CAIs do not appear to have any additive effects to oral CAIs.[4]

References

1. Gabelt BT, Kaufman PL. Cholinergic drugs. In: Netland PA, Allen RC, eds. *Glaucoma Medical Therapy*. San Francisco, CA: Foundation of the American Academy of Ophthalmology; 1999:77-97.
2. Allen RC. Carbonic anhydrase inhibitors. In: Netland PA, Allen RC, eds. *Glaucoma Medical Therapy*. San Francisco, CA: Foundation of the American Academy of Ophthalmology; 1999:99-111.
3. Lichter PR. Reducing side effects of carbonic anhydrase inhibitors. *Ophthalmology*. 1981;88:266-269.
4. Rosenberg LF, Krupin T, Tang LQ, Hong PH, Ruderman JH. Combination of systemic acetazolamide and topical dorzalamide in reducing intraocular pressure and aqueous humor formation. *Ophthalmology*. 1998;105:88-93.

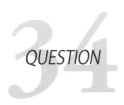

HOW CAN I IMPROVE PATIENT ADHERENCE?

Silvia Orengo-Nania, MD

The terms *adherence* and *compliance* are seen often in the medical literature and used interchangeably to define the extent of agreement between the prescribed medical regimen and actual patient practice. In general, poor adherence to medications accounts for substantial worsening of disease, death, and increased health care costs in the United States with a resultant cost of approximately $100 billion a year.[1] Both indirect and direct ways of measuring adherence with a medication can be used. Direct methods include blood or urine levels of the medication or its metabolite or direct observation. Indirect methods include asking the patient whether he or she took his or her medication, assessing the clinical response, performing pill counts, obtaining refill rates, and electronic medication monitors.

Adherence is critical in managing patients with glaucoma, but not always easily measured. Several studies have shown that the lower the intraocular pressure (IOP), the less likely the patient will be to progress.[2–5] We also suspect that fluctuation in IOP can lead to visual field progression. Therefore, if the patient does not take the medication daily and as prescribed by the doctor, there can be worsening of the disease, leading to visual impairment. Adequate treatment of glaucoma requires a high level of compliance to therapy.[6] However, studies have shown that nonadherence with ocular hypotensive medication regimens is common among our patients, occurring among approximately 5% to 80%.[7]

To improve patient adherence, we must recognize the risk factors for nonadherence. These can be divided into patient-centered issues, situational issues, medication regimen–related issues, and provider-related issues. Patient-related issues include poor understanding of the disease (by the patient and family members), poor cognitive ability, literacy level, and poor general health. Situational issues include erratic work schedules, shift work, busy lifestyle, and major life events. Multiple studies have shown that the dosing regimen is important for compliance. Severity of disease is also a predictive factor for adherence; the more severe the disease, the more adherent to treatment.[8]

Gedde SJ, ed. *Curbside Consultation in Glaucoma:*
49 Clinical Questions, Second Edition (pp 159–161)
© 2015 Taylor & Francis Group

As the number of medicines increases and the number of applications increases, adherence decreases. Provider-related issues include the cost of medication (which can play an important role in nonadherence, especially if the patient is taking multiple medications) and the provider's ability to gain the patient's trust and commitment to follow the prescribed regimen.

Some of the ways in which we can try to improve our patients' adherence to glaucoma therapy include the following: increasing patient education, improving our doctor-patient relationships, facilitating access for follow-up appointments and testing, simplifying dosing regimens, instructing our patients in drop installation techniques and confirming proficiency during follow-up visits, and using reminder mechanisms.[9] Patient and family education regarding the disease is critical to ensure patient understanding about the need to take the medications exactly as prescribed and to engender patient cooperation. Because glaucoma is an asymptomatic disease that is slowly progressive, without a good understanding of the potential outcome of poor adherence, patients will not commit to maintaining the prescribed regimen. Patient education can be done one-on-one with the doctor, which has an added bonus of improving the patient-doctor relationship and increasing trust in the doctor. However, this cannot always be achieved in a busy practice. Another way to increase patient education is to provide our patients with printed literature on glaucoma and the importance of compliance. This can be achieved with a multitude of pamphlets published by academic as well as pharmaceutical sources. Office personnel can also provide valuable educational information on a personal level with the aid of pamphlets and educational videos.

To address some of the other patient-related issues for nonadherence, the doctor and office staff can create handouts for the patients that describe the medication by the color of the top rather than name and give times for applications that coincide with daily activities. Attention to dosing regimens can eliminate some medication-related risk factors to nonadherence. These regimens should be made as simple as possible with the fewest number of medications and dosing intervals as possible. To minimize the cost-related pressures for nonadherence, we can facilitate procurement of medication assistance programs through the pharmaceutical companies or proceed with laser or surgical treatment. To prevent other provider-related issues for nonadherence, we must be available to see our patients as often as necessary to give the patients a sense of importance and urgency in controlling their disease. We must take an active role in inquiring about compliance by asking our patients about missed doses and help our patients create approaches that facilitate increased adherence. New devices are also available such as electronic reminders, phone call reminders, and electronic monitoring of drop use that we can use to monitor adherence. Another personal technique that I found very useful in demonstrating how strict adherence is necessary is to have the patient stop his or her medications the day before coming to see me and note how high the IOP is with just one day of not using the medication.

Summary

One of the most important aspects of glaucoma management is ensuring that our patients understand the importance of consistent medical management of their disease. We must take an active role in educating patients and ensuring that they follow the regimen prescribed. If this goal is not achieved, then we have failed in our mission of preventing blindness in our patients with glaucoma. In my clinic, I give new patients a concise simplified lecture on the disease and a pamphlet to bring home for themselves, as well as their family, to read. For the next few visits, we discuss adherence and side effects of the medications. Just as a patient is becoming complacent, I ask him or her to stop the medication the day before the next visit to increase his or her awareness of the importance of compliance. I also make sure that the patient has more than enough refills to prevent lapses in therapy. If all of this fails, then we begin the discussion on the surgical management of glaucoma, which essentially removes adherence as a factor in the management of this disease.

References

1. Osterber L, Bhalcshke T. Adherence to medication. *N Engl J Med*. 2005;353:487-497.
2. Epstein DL, Drug JH Jr, Hertzmark E, et al. A long-term clinical trial of timolol therapy versus no treatment in the management of glaucoma suspects. *Ophthalmology*. 1989;96:1460-1467.
3. Kass MA, Gordon MO, Hoff MR, et al. Topical timolol administration reduces the incidence of glaucomatous damage in ocular hypertensive individuals: a randomized, double-masked, long-term clinical trial. *Arch Ophthalmol*. 1989;107:1590-1598.
4. Kass MA, Heuer EDK, Higginbotham EJ, et al; Ocular Hypertension Treatment Study Group. The Ocular Hypertension Treatment Study: a randomized trial determines that topical ocular hypotensive medication delays or prevents the onset of primary open-angle glaucoma. *Arch Ophthalmol*. 2002;120:701-713.
5. Musch DE, Gillespie BW, Lichter PR, et al; GIGTS Study Investigators Visual field progression in the Collaborative Initial Glaucoma Treatment Study: the impact of treatment and other baseline factors. *Ophthalmology*. 2009;116:200-2001.
6. American Academy of Ophthalmology. *Preferred Practice Pattern: Primary Open-Angle Glaucoma*. San Francisco, CA: American Academy of Ophthalmology; 2003:13.
7. Olthoff CM. Schouten JS, van de Borne BW, Webers CA. Noncompliance with ocular hypertensive treatment in patients with glaucoma or ocular hypertension: an evidence-based review. *Ophthalmology*. 2005;112:953-961.
8. Ung C, Shang E, Alfaro T, et al. Glaucoma severity and medication adherence in a county hospital population. *Ophthalmology*. 2013;120:1150-1157.
9. Tsai JC. Medication adherence in glaucoma: approaches for optimizing patient compliance. *Curr Opin Ophthalmol*. 2006;17:190-195.

SECTION V

LASER AND INCISIONAL GLAUCOMA SURGERY

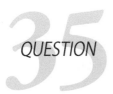

IS SELECTIVE LASER TRABECULOPLASTY A REPEATABLE PROCEDURE? WHEN SHOULD I USE IT?

Brian A. Francis, MD, MS

Background

Laser trabeculoplasty (LTP) has traditionally been employed as an adjunct to maximum tolerated medical therapy to lower intraocular pressure (IOP) in patients with open-angle glaucoma (OAG). The original procedure was described using an argon laser (major peaks at 488 and 514 nm). The Glaucoma Laser Trial showed that in patients with newly diagnosed OAG, argon laser trabeculoplasty (ALT) was at least as effective as initial treatment with timolol maleate 0.5%, even after 7 years.[1] However, ALT produces tissue disruption and coagulation damage to the trabecular meshwork, possibly contributing to the limited effectiveness of retreatment.[2] This, coupled with the fact that most patients ended up receiving medications eventually, led to the failure of acceptance of ALT as primary glaucoma therapy. Most physicians in the United States maintained the algorithm of medication first, then LTP, and finally filtration surgery. However, with the advent of newer laser platforms, this paradigm may be changing.

Selective laser trabeculoplasty (SLT), approved by the US Food and Drug Administration (FDA) in March 2001, consists of a 532-nm, frequency-doubled, Q-switched Nd:YAG laser. It results in the selective absorption of energy by pigmented cells in the trabecular meshwork and spares adjacent cells and tissues from thermal energy damage. Compared with ALT, each SLT pulse delivers less than 0.1% total energy and is 8 orders of magnitude shorter in duration.

Patient Selection

SLT can theoretically be used in any patient with OAG or ocular hypertension (OHT) in whom glaucoma medications are considered. It can be used as an initial therapy instead of medications, as

Gedde SJ, ed. *Curbside Consultation in Glaucoma:*
49 Clinical Questions, Second Edition (pp 165–168)
© 2015 Taylor & Francis Group

a replacement for medications in medically controlled glaucoma, or as an adjunct to medically un-controlled glaucoma. In general, the procedure works best when used with fewer glaucoma medi-cations. Let's start with one end of the treatment spectrum with OHT and follow through to uncontrolled glaucoma after failed glaucoma surgery.

I will offer SLT to patients with high-risk OHT (as defined by the Ocular Hypertension Treat-ment Study) in whom I would recommend medical treatment. Similarly, I think it is appropriate as a first-line treatment in patients with newly diagnosed glaucoma. The SLT/MED study by Katz and colleagues[3] was a multicenter, randomized trial that compared initial laser vs medical treat-ment of OAG. The results indicated a similar response in IOP reduction with SLT and medical therapy, which consisted primarily of prostaglandin use. These results were supported by Nagar et al,[4] who found in a randomized trial of patients with OAG that 360-degree treatment was most effective with SLT and resulted in similar reductions in IOP compared with latanaprost. Thus, a reasonable expectation for lowering IOP is in the 30% range from an untreated baseline.

Perhaps the largest group of patients that we see clinically is those who are controlled with one or more glaucoma medications. We prospectively studied this patient population and the ability to reduce medications after SLT while still maintaining target IOP.[5] We found that medications could be reduced or eliminated in approximately 87% of patients at 1 year. Thus, I offer SLT treat-ment to patients with OAG who are medically controlled and may wish to reduce their medication burden.

Finally, there is the group of patients with uncontrolled IOP who take the maximum tolerated glaucoma medications. SLT has proven helpful as an adjunct in these cases, but in general, the more medications that are being used, the less IOP reduction one can expect from SLT. In general, I would expect a 15% to 20% lowering of IOP when SLT is added to a medication and incremen-tally less with higher numbers of medications. However, at times, a patient with several medica-tions can have quite large IOP reductions with laser.

The effects of SLT have also been studied in patients with failed glaucoma filtration surgery such as trabeculectomy[6] and the newer angle-based minimally invasive glaucoma surgeries.[7] The efficacy in these patients is limited, and therefore I only offer it if patients are not good candidates for further incisional surgery.

Selective Laser Trabeculoplasty Procedure

The Q-switched, frequency-doubled, 532-nm Nd:YAG laser (Lumenis Selecta SLT Laser; Lu-menis, Inc, Santa Clara, California) is used with a wavelength of 532 nm and pulse duration of 3 ns. I pretreat with apraclonidine 1.0% or brimonidine 0.1% to 0.2%. For patient comfort, I also treat with a drop of a topical nonsteroidal anti-inflammatory drug (NSAID) and give the patient a prescription for this to use 2 to 3 times a day if needed. Most patients do not require it. Initially, our protocol was to apply 50 spots over 180 degrees and that evolved into approximately 100 con-tiguous spots over 360 degrees. Currently, I use a greater number of spots, such that they overlap, and with a lower power level. My starting power is approximately 0.5 to 0.6 mJ, titrating so that the small cavitation energy bubbles are rarely seen. The energy delivery can vary depending on the age of the laser or how much it is handled and transported. I find that newer lasers and those that are not moved constantly are more efficient in energy delivery and require lower powers. I typically perform 130 to 150 spots over 360 degrees of trabecular meshwork.

It is critical to target the correct tissue during treatment. Gonioscopy should be performed prior to the laser to identify angle opening. If the angle is narrow, pilocarpine can be used preoperatively, or a light may be shined in the contralateral eye to constrict the pupil. The patient can also be in-structed to look toward the treating mirror, which will rotate the angle into better view. In a narrow angle, do not mistake a pigmented Schwalbe's line for trabecular meshwork. In a deep angle with less pigment, do not mistakenly treat ciliary body band instead of trabecular meshwork. If the landmarks are not clear in a narrow angle, I find it helpful to use compression gonioscopy prior to laser to identify them. In a poorly pigmented angle, it is helpful to view the inferior angle, as there may be more pigment in the inferior trabecular meshwork. Occasionally, applying pressure with the laser gonio lens (such as a 3-mirror Goldmann lens) will cause blood to reflux into Schlemm's canal and assist in identifying the trabecular meshwork.

After laser, I check the IOP 1 hour later to detect significant IOP spikes and treat them accordingly. Depending on the severity of glaucoma damage, I either stop the medication at the time of laser or continue medications and begin to decrease them at the 1-month visit. Since the method of action is a biological response, it may take 3 months or longer to see a significant response.

Repeat Selective Laser Trabeculoplasty

Because of the very short pulse duration of SLT (compared with thermal relaxation time of the tissue), adjacent tissues do not absorb the laser energy, and the spread of heat damage is minimized. This difference in tissue effect (compared with ALT) allows for the potential of retreatment with SLT. Retreatment is usually performed when an initial treatment has been successful, but the effect wears off over time. However, it is sometimes done when the initial response is not enough to reach target IOP levels. In my clinical practice, the first scenario is usually the case in retreatment. Studies have shown that the IOP-lowering response of the repeat laser is comparable to the first treatment.[8] The lasers in this trial were separated by at least 6 months.

Practically speaking, if the IOP is successfully controlled for 1 year or more, repeat SLT should be considered. There is a limit in clinical practice to how many times the procedure can be successfully treated, and this likely varies with the individual patient. At some point, the IOP will not decrease with multiple repeated treatments and may in fact rise.

Summary

SLT is effective in the initial, adjunctive, and repeat treatment of OAG. The latter scenario includes patients who have had an initial successful treatment with 360-degree SLT, with the effect wearing off over time. This may offer an advantage over ALT, in which repeated treatments result in progressive damage to the trabecular meshwork and diminishing success. The difference may be attributable to the selective targeting of pigmented cells with SLT and the lack of coagulative damage to the outflow tissues. Patient selection and proper technique, including targeting the appropriate tissue, is important to maximize success.

References

1. The Glaucoma Laser Trial Research Group. The Glaucoma Laser Trial (GLT) and glaucoma laser trial follow-up study, seven-year results. *Am J Ophthalmol.* 1995;120:718-731.
2. Grayson DK, Camras CB, Podos SM, Lustgarten JS. Long-term reduction of intraocular pressure after repeat argon laser trabeculoplasty. *Am J Ophthalmol.* 1988;106:312-321.
3. Katz LJ, Steinmann WC, Kabir Z, Molineaux J, Wizov SS, Marcellino G. Selective laser trabeculoplasty versus medical therapy as initial treatment of glaucoma. *J Glaucoma.* 2012;21(7):460-468.
4. Nagar M, Ogunyomade A, O'Brart DP, et al. A randomized, prospective study comparing selective laser trabeculoplasty with latanoprost for the control of intraocular pressure in ocular hypertension and open angle glaucoma. *Br J Ophthalmol.* 2005;89:1413-1417.

5. Francis BA, Ianchulev T, Schofield JK, Minckler DS. Selective laser trabeculoplasty as a replacement for medical therapy in open angle glaucoma. *Am J Ophthalmol.* 2005;140(3):524-525.
6. Francis BA, Traudt B, Enright J, Herzog D, Chopra V, Azen S. Selective laser trabeculoplasty (SLT) after failed trabeculectomy in open angle glaucoma. *J Clin Exp Ophthalmol.* 2011;8(2):1-4.
7. Toteberg-Harms M, Rhee DJ. Selective laser trabeculoplasty following failed combined phacoemulsification cataract extraction and ab interno trabeculectomy. *Am J Ophthalmol.* 2013;156:936-940.
8. Hong BK, Winer JC, Martone JF, Wand M, Altman B, Shields B. Repeat selective laser trabeculoplasty. *J Glaucoma.* 2009;18:180-183.

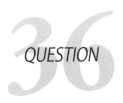

36

WHEN SHOULD I PERFORM A PROPHYLACTIC LASER IRIDOTOMY?

Martin Wand, MD

For the purposes of this question within the context of angle closure glaucoma (ACG), we will be discussing mainly primary ACG (PACG).

There are few instances in medicine when the indications for a procedure are as clear-cut as a prophylactic laser peripheral iridotomy (LPI) as in the fellow eye of a patient who has already had acute ACG in one eye. Since ACG is a bilateral disorder, the chances of acute ACG in the fellow eye are 40% over 5 years.[1] With the relative safety and ease of LPI, this is an easy and sound decision. An obvious exception to this general rule is if the fellow eye is already pseudophakic and in no danger of ACG.

Furthermore, in a patient who presents with a history consistent with intermittent ACG and on examination the anterior chamber angles are deemed narrow enough to be spontaneously closable on gonioscopy and the eye shows signs of previous bouts of ACG, prophylactic LPI is indicated in both eyes. The findings suggestive of previous bouts of acute ACG include sector iris atrophy, an irregularly and permanently dilated pupil, glaukomflecken, and/or peripheral anterior synechiae (PAS). What constitutes a narrow spontaneously closable angle is a more difficult question that will be addressed later.

Another indication for prophylactic LPI is in a patient who has open-angle glaucoma (OAG) in whom laser trabeculoplasty (LTP) is being considered but in whom the anterior chamber angles are not readily visible through the optics of the laser delivery system. With the independent slit lamp's greater mobility and the use of gonioscopy lenses that have a smaller surface diameter to allow simultaneous compression of the angle, it is often possible to visualize the functional trabecular meshwork in an eye with open yet narrow angles, especially when the eye looks toward the goniolens mirror. However, with the less mobile optical system of the laser delivery system and the use of larger diameter Goldmann or similar lenses, angle structures may not be readily visible for LTP in such eyes. In these patients needing LTP, they are often older, and there is often some

Gedde SJ, ed. *Curbside Consultation in Glaucoma:
49 Clinical Questions, Second Edition* (pp 169–173)
© 2015 Taylor & Francis Group

component of relative pupillary block; an LPI will relieve the pupillary block component and thereby may flatten the iris enough to allow adequate visualization for LTP. In the past, it has been recommended to apply the argon laser beam on the convex peripheral iris to contract it and allow visualization of the anterior chamber angle. While this peripheral iridoplasty can indeed open the angle, this may also lead to more inflammation and could result in PAS. A prophylactic LPI is easier and safer in this situation.

The most common situation when a prophylactic LPI is indicated is an asymptomatic patient found to have narrow angles on routine examination. If appositional closure is present (ie, if angle structures are not visible on gonioscopy except with compression), an LPI may decrease the risk of subsequent PAS formation and intraocular pressure (IOP) elevation.

A prophylactic LPI may also be considered when the anterior chamber angles are very narrow on gonioscopy and deemed to be spontaneously closable because the angle generally becomes narrower with increasing age. The relative safety of LPI makes it justifiable for such a patient who will not have adequate ophthalmic care in the future—for example, a patient who is moving to a remote part of the world, if the physical and/or mental health of the patient are known to be rapidly deteriorating, or in cases of inability to get the patient back to care.

One other clinical condition, although not PACG, should be mentioned here for which a prophylactic LPI may be indicated. In pigmentary dispersion syndrome (PDS), there may be reverse pupillary block causing the posterior pigmented iris surface to rub against the lens zonules, resulting in pigment dispersion and a secondary glaucoma in some patients. Through participation of the American Glaucoma Society members, we have looked at patients with PDS in whom one eye had a prophylactic LPI. Although there was a mean 4-mm Hg lower IOP in the treated eye at the end of 2 years, the results may have been biased because the treated eyes had a higher baseline IOP, and our patients were older than the typical patient with PDS.[2] Lacking a definitive study, I would do an LPI in a young (< 40 years) patient with PDS who has substantial concavity of the peripheral iris confirming the presence of reverse pupillary block.

The holy grail of ACG is to have a test that will reliably predict whether an eye will develop ACG so that a prophylactic LPI can be performed. Unfortunately, in a nutshell, there is as yet no such test. With the advent of ultrasound biomicroscopy (UBM) and anterior segment optical coherence tomography (ASOCT), although the view of angle structures may not be as clear as with UBM, we now have 2 techniques of objectively imaging the anterior chamber angle, undistorted by compression, light-induced miosis, or accommodation. Many types of secondary ACGs have been elucidated with these techniques, and even physiologic anatomic changes associated with angle closure can now be observed in real time. Unfortunately, both instruments are expensive, are generally not available to practitioners, and have their own limitations; most important, no studies yet have confirmed that either technology is better than gonioscopy in predicting if or when ACG might occur. At the present time, the decision to do a prophylactic LPI must still be based on clinical judgment and experience, as well as gonioscopy. It is also of significance that gonioscopy has been shown to be woefully underperformed in this country. While the American Academy of Ophthalmology's Preferred Practice Pattern recommends doing gonioscopy on all patients presenting with glaucoma to differentiate ACG from OAG, less than 50% of all patients have had a gonioscopic examination during the 4 to 5 years prior to having glaucoma surgery, including LPIs.[3]

While there are no hard data to prove this, prophylactic LPIs probably are also underperformed in this country. From the latest Medicare data available (2004), the number of LPIs performed in the United States has hovered below 80,000 per year since 1994.[4] At the same time, there has been a significant increase in the number of LTPs performed. The analogy of LPI and appendectomy is appropriate in this context. A good general surgeon will remove a number of noninflamed appendixes, just as a good ophthalmic surgeon will perform a number of LPIs in eyes that might never have developed ACG.

Needless to say, there is perhaps equal danger in overdoing LPIs, especially when they are not indicated, since LPI is not a totally benign procedure. Among the potential complications are corneal burns, iris bleeding, iritis, posterior synechiae, elevated IOPs, cataract formation, imperforate iridotomies, and rare cases of retinal detachment. One would hope that there are no clinicians who would knowingly do an LPI for which there are no indications. The only solution possible, at best, is better education of both the clinicians (on ethics as well as diagnostics) and patients (to seek second opinions when there is any doubt).

There are many ways to perform an LPI. The technique I will describe has evolved based on the optical properties of Nd:YAG lasers as well as experience in doing LPIs for over 30 years. Since the advent of the Nd:YAG laser in 1981, I have not performed any argon LPIs. Many still advocate argon LPI either as a single-laser modality of treatment or combined with Nd:YAG lasers. I will confine myself to Nd:YAG lasers as my single-treatment modality, but I will make a few comments on pretreatment with the argon laser. The major cited reasons are to coagulate iris stromal blood vessels to prevent bleeding; to thin thicker, especially darker, irides; and to tense the iris to allow easier penetration with the Nd:YAG laser. Argon laser pretreatment could coagulate vessels on the iris surface as well as nonvisible deeper stromal vessels. However, in practice, we can almost always see blood vessels in the iris, so they are easy to avoid, and if one preferentially places laser burns in an iris crypt, if there is one in the appropriate location, usually no vessels are at the base of crypts. In addition, most iris bleeding is of a transient and minor nature that can be easily controlled with moderate pressure on the treating gonioscopy lens for 1 minute or so. Argon laser pretreatment can be helpful in eyes with thicker, dark irides. However, even in such eyes, using the Nd:YAG laser, there have been only a few occasions where I have had to let the iris debris settle for a few minutes and then continue treatment in the resulting thinner stoma to penetrate the iris.

The argon laser produces a coherent laser beam, and macula burns have been reported with this laser—hence the admonition to keep the argon laser beam angled toward the periphery using an Abraham lens with a peripheral magnifying button. With either Abraham lens with the peripheral button or central button (my preference), the Nd:YAG laser beam has 24 degrees of convergence so that approximately 4 mm beyond the plane of focus, the power of the laser is below the retinal injury threshold, so it would be difficult, if not impossible, to cause a retinal burn with a Nd:YAG LPI. In addition, as you will recall from doing Nd:YAG laser capsulotomies, proper focusing of the Nd:YAG laser is critical; when the Nd:YAG laser is slightly out of focus or not perpendicular to the surface being treated, there is no effect on the capsule. For these reasons, I use only the center-button Abraham lens and I have the patient look straight ahead and I adjust the laser so that the HeNe aiming beam is perpendicular to the iris surface through the center of the Abraham lens. The zone of photodisruption for the Nd:YAG laser is slightly anterior to its focal plane. Some of the newer Nd:YAG lasers can be set slightly retrofocused, but if on the initial burst there is a crater formed on the iris surface without penetration with your Nd:YAG laser, you may have to retrofocus slightly more on the iris. However, if you retrofocus too much, you can disrupt the posterior iris pigment layer without stromal penetration. So transillumination is not an indication of a successful LPI with the Nd:YAG laser, as it is with the argon LPIs and incisional peripheral iridectomies; a gush of aqueous with pigment granules signifies penetration with the Nd:YAG laser.

My Nd:YAG laser settings are 5.0 mJ at 2 pulses/burst, but I am sure that many other settings would perform equally well. I always try to use an iris crypt if there is one in or near the location I want, which is in the 3- or 9-o'clock position. The angle is most shallow superior and deeper nasally than temporally, so I usually do them nasally. Traditionally, surgical peripheral iridotomies (PIs) have been done superiorly, and by extension, argon LPIs and Nd:YAG LPIs have also been done superiorly. I can think of only one other reason why surgical PIs and LPIs might have been done initially in the superior quadrant: possible glare from an exposed PI certainly made it seem logical to place the PI beneath the upper lid. However, experience has shown the contrary. For the past 30+ years, I have done my LPIs in the horizontal axis without a single subsequent complaint of dysphotopsia, but we continue to learn of dysphotopsia in patients who have had superior PIs. Murphy and Trope[5] reported that superior PIs did not cause any visual symptoms if they were fully covered by the upper lid or if they were fully exposed by lifting the upper lid completely away from PI. At a meeting of the Nassau County Ophthalmologic Society in the early 1990s, I gave a talk on ACG and mentioned that I did not know the cause of visual symptoms after some superior LPIs. One of the ophthalmologists at the meeting, Joel Weintraub, told me that he thought this was due to the tear meniscus at the upper lid edge margin. If the tear meniscus straddled the superior PI, this would result in a base-up high-minus prism that could cause the diplopia; this was subsequently reported.[6] This also explains why when the lid is lifted up, thereby eliminating the tear meniscus over the PI, the visual symptoms resolve. Recently, Vera et al[7] performed a prospective, randomized, single-masked, paired study in which 153 consecutive patients had a superior LPI in one eye and a temporal LPI in the fellow eye. They found that 11.1% with superior LPIs had dysphotopsia vs 3.3% with temporal LPIs ($P = .007$). They also pointed out that the smaller YAG laser PI, compared with the larger argon laser PI, would result in greater light diffraction.

There are good reasons, besides a lower incidence of dysphotopsia, to place the LPIs in the horizontal axis. The angle is most narrow superiorly, and the frequent presence of a superior corneal arcus makes visualization of the superior peripheral iris difficult as well as more likely to result in corneal endothelial damage. Furthermore, it is easier to have the patient look slightly sideways than to look far downward. In the rare event of an iris bleed, blood from a superior PI would cover the visual axis, whereas blood from a PI temporally or nasally would not be noticed by the patient.

After more than 30 years of crusading, I am pleased to note at talks around the country that at straw polls of audiences, the number of ophthalmologists who perform LPIs in the horizontal axis has increased from none to almost 50%. However, I am also disappointed to report that according to the 2007 AAO Practicing Ophthalmologist Curriculum for ACG,[8] the study guide for maintaining the certification process, the Academy is still not willing to commit to recommending placing LPIs in the horizontal axis. They will commit only to "plac[ing] the PI anywhere except where it might straddle the upper lid margin," which nevertheless represents progress from the previous recommendation of placing LPIs superiorly!

Summary

A prophylactic LPI should be performed in the fellow eye of patients with an acute episode of angle closure. Eyes with gonioscopically confirmed narrow angles and symptoms and findings consistent with previous bouts of ACG should be treated as well. An iridotomy should also be considered in eyes with angles gonioscopically narrow enough to be deemed spontaneously closable and possibly in eyes with PDS of young patients with documented concavity of the iris with pigment dispersion.

References

1. Weinreb RN, Friedman DS, eds. *Angle Closure and Angle Closure Glaucoma*. The Hague, the Netherlands: Kugler; 2006.
2. Reistad CE, Shields MB, Campbell DG, et al. The influence of peripheral iridotomy on the intraocular pressure course in patients with pigmentary glaucoma. *J Glaucoma*. 2005;14:255-259.
3. Coleman AL, Yu F, Evans SJ. Use of gonioscopy in Medicare beneficiaries before glaucoma surgery. *J Glaucoma*. 2006;15:486-493.

4. Rivera AH, Brown RH, Anderson DR. Laser iridotomy vs surgical iridectomy. Have the indications changed? *Arch Ophth*. 1985;103(9):1350-1354.
5. Murphy PH, Trope GE. Monocular blurring; a complication of YAG laser iridotomy. *Ophthalmology*. 1991;98:1539-1542.
6. Weintraub J, Berke SJ. Blurring after iridotomy. *Ophthalmology*. 1992;99:479-480.
7. Vera M, Vanessa I, Naqui A, Ahmed I. Dysphotopsia following temporal versus superior laser peripheral iridotomies. *Am J Ophthalmol*. 2014;157(5):929-935.
8. American Academy of Ophthalmology, San Francisco, CA, 2007.

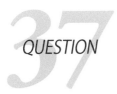

WHEN IS LASER IRIDOPLASTY USED?

Alon Skaat, MD and
Jeffrey M. Liebmann, MD

The angle closure glaucomas are a diverse group of disorders characterized by iridotrabecular apposition, trabecular injury and dysfunction, elevated intraocular pressure (IOP), glaucomatous optic neuropathy, and visual field loss. Although angle closure can develop from a variety of causes, almost all cases of primary angle closure have a component of relative pupillary block. Since laser iridotomy successfully eliminates the relative pupillary block component of the angle closure process, it should be performed in all eyes with primary angle closure.

Argon laser peripheral iridoplasty (ALPI) is a laser surgical technique designed to reduce or eliminate iridotrabecular contact when laser iridotomy fails to open an appositionally closed angle (ie, a non-pupillary block mechanism) or when laser iridotomy is not possible.[1-4] The procedure involves the placement of laser applications in the iris periphery to both compact the iris stroma and contract it away from the angle. Careful attention to the differential diagnosis of angle closure remains the key to the early detection of eyes that may fail to respond to laser iridotomy or may develop recurrent angle closure. It should be noted that synechial angle closure (peripheral anterior synechiae, [PAS]) cannot be altered by iridoplasty.

Persistent iridotrabecular apposition following successful laser iridotomy and resolution of a pupillary block typically occurs due to an angle closure process that originates posterior to the iris plane. This can occur at the level of the ciliary body, lens, or from forces within the posterior segment. Plateau iris configuration or syndrome, lens-induced angle closure (intumescence, subluxation, or dislocation), or posterior segment processes (malignant glaucoma syndromes, central retinal vein occlusion, scleral buckling, extensive pan-retinal photocoagulation, or adverse reaction to certain systemic medications [eg, topiramate]) are potential causes of a non-pupillary block angle closure mechanism.

ALPI is generally indicated to reduce or eliminate residual or persistent iridotrabecular apposition in eyes with a functioning iridotomy. An iridotomy can only be deemed patent by visualizing

Gedde SJ, ed. *Curbside Consultation in Glaucoma:*
49 Clinical Questions, Second Edition (pp 175–178)
© 2015 Taylor & Francis Group

the anterior lens capsule through it or if a lack of iris convexity can be demonstrated by imaging the anterior segment. Retroillumination alone is not sufficient to determine iridotomy patency. Any residual pupillary block will eventually overcome the effect of a perfectly performed iridoplasty.

Specific Indications for Argon Laser Peripheral Iridoplasty

RESIDUAL APPOSITIONAL CLOSURE FOLLOWING LASER IRIDOTOMY

Pupillary block is the cause of iridotrabecular apposition in the vast majority of eyes with primary angle closure and is relieved by laser iridotomy. ALPI is indicated if indentation gonioscopy confirms the presence of persistent iridotrabecular apposition. It is not indicated if indentation reveals only synechial closure (PAS) without residual apposition. Plateau iris configuration or syndrome is the most common cause of recurrent or persistent iridotrabecular apposition and responds well to iridoplasty. Eyes with a shallow anterior segment due to enlargement or anterior subluxation (eg, zonular laxity due to exfoliation syndrome) of the crystalline lens often respond less well.

ACUTE ANGLE CLOSURE IN THE PRESENCE OF A PATENT LASER IRIDOTOMY

Recurrent angle closure following successful iridotomy is consistent with a non-pupillary angle closure block mechanism. ALPI can be performed to break the acute attack (described next) or widen the angle after the attack has been broken.

ACUTE ANGLE CLOSURE WHERE LASER IRIDOTOMY IS NOT POSSIBLE DUE TO HAZY MEDIA

Treatment of acute angle closure (acute angle closure glaucoma or acute angle closure glaucoma "attack") is a reduction of IOP and a reversal of the anatomic configuration that led to the attack. Since many patients are in pain and experience emesis, rapid intervention is usually warranted. In cases where medical therapy fails to reduce the IOP or laser iridotomy cannot be performed due to hazy media, ALPI can be used to break the acute attack, lower IOP, provide an interval for medical therapy to become effective, and facilitate laser iridotomy through clear media. For many eyes with lens-related angle closure, ALPI can provide an interval for cessation of inflammation and lower IOP prior to cataract surgery. Even if the attack is broken, iridotomy should be performed as soon as possible to eliminate any relative pupillary block that remains.

RECURRENT APPOSITIONAL CLOSURE AFTER IRIDOTOMY AND IRIDOPLASTY

Eyes that require ALPI often have unusual angle configurations or ocular anatomy. Gonioscopy should be repeated on a periodic basis, and progressive angle narrowing with recurrent iridotrabecular apposition may indicate the need for repeat iridoplasty years after the initial treatment. Many of these eyes respond well to cataract surgery, which typically widens the anterior chamber angle.

PRIOR TO LASER TRABECULOPLASTY WHEN THE ANGLE REMAINS ANATOMICALLY NARROW FOLLOWING IRIDOTOMY

In some patients, an anatomically narrow angle makes laser trabeculoplasty technically difficult. ALPI can be used to widen the angle in the few individuals in whom better laser lens positioning or appropriate direction of gaze fails to provide an adequate gonioscopic view. These eyes often have an angle that is ultimately too narrow for laser trabeculoplasty and are at increased risk for the development of peripheral anterior synechiae. Other forms of glaucoma therapy, often combined with lens extraction, may be better alternatives for these eyes.

INDICATIONS OTHER THAN GLAUCOMA

Laser iridoplasty may also be used to contract the iris away from other intraocular structures or implants obstructing the visual axis or alter pupillary configuration in eyes with complex anterior segment anatomy. The placement of the laser iridoplasty applications varies based on the particular patient. These indications are infrequently encountered.

Laser Surgical Technique

Successful laser iridoplasty depends on accurate placement of the laser applications at the peripheral iris.[1-3] Each application should be large (500-micron spot size), have a long duration (0.5 seconds), and use relatively low power (200 to 500 milliwatts, depending on iris pigmentation). Preoperative pilocarpine should be administered to immobilize the pupil and bring the peripheral iris into view. An Abraham-type lens facilitates aiming of the laser beam, which should pass partly through the limbus to make certain that the application is peripheral. The immediate laser effect is contraction of the iris toward the center of the application. A total of 24 to 30 applications should be placed circumferentially and visible blood vessels avoided. Excessive laser applications may cause chronic inflammation or iris ischemia, resulting in an enlarged or minimally reactive pupil (Urrets-Zavalia syndrome).[5] Postoperative treatment with a topical corticosteroid 4 times daily for 4 days is usually sufficient to minimize intraocular inflammation. Healed laser iridoplasty applications are often visible in the extreme periphery.

Summary

Iridoplasty is a useful technique to widen the anterior chamber angle in the appropriate clinical setting. Although the technique is well established, care must be taken to avoid complications such as iris ischemia, peripheral anterior synechiae, and corneal injury. However, meticulous placement of the laser applications and careful patient selection provide for rewarding results in these difficult angle closure eyes.

References

1. Ritch R, Liebmann JM. Argon laser peripheral iridoplasty. *Ophthalmic Surg Lasers*. 1996;27:289-300.
2. Liebmann JM, Ritch R. Laser surgery for angle closure glaucoma. *Semin Ophthalmol*. 2002;17(2):84-91.

3. Ritch R, Tham CC, Lam DS. Argon laser peripheral iridoplasty (ALPI): an update. *Surv Ophthalmol.* 2007;52:279-288.
4. Ritch R. Argon laser treatment for medically unresponsive attacks of angle-closure glaucoma. *Am J Ophthalmol.* 1982;94:197-204.
5. Espana EM, Ioannidis A, Tello C, Liebmann JM, Foster P, Ritch R. Urrets-Zavalia syndrome as a complication of argon laser peripheral iridoplasty. *Br J Ophthalmol.* 2007;91:427-429.

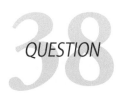

WHEN SHOULD I PERFORM INCISIONAL GLAUCOMA SURGERY? WHICH PROCEDURE SHOULD I CHOOSE?

Joseph F. Panarelli, MD

When Should I Perform Surgery?

The decision to perform incisional glaucoma surgery is not an easy one. Surgery has traditionally been reserved for patients who are progressing or are deemed likely to progress despite maximally tolerated medical and/or laser therapy. It is at this point that the risk of continuing to observe outweighs the risks of performing surgery. Doctors, as well as patients, are often reluctant to go to the operating room early during the course of treatment despite the results of landmark studies such as the Collaborative Initial Glaucoma Treatment Study (CIGTS), which have challenged the traditional therapeutic approach. The CIGTS study found that lowering intraocular pressure (IOP) with initial filtering surgery is as effective as medical therapy for slowing progression of visual field loss. In fact, patients with more advanced visual field loss (mean deviation worse than −10 dB) actually did better with initial surgery compared with those who were initially treated with medication.[1-4] Surgically treated patients likely benefit from less diurnal IOP fluctuation, lower peak pressures, and a lower mean IOP. In the Moorfields Primary Treatment Trial (PTT), patients who underwent trabeculectomy had a mean IOP of 14.5 mm Hg at 5 years compared with 18.5 mm Hg for those patients treated with either medication or laser therapy. In addition, there was a higher rate of success for the surgical group that was sustained throughout the 5 years of follow-up.[5,6] Neither the Moorfields PTT nor CIGTS studies found any significant difference in the mean loss of visual acuity between the medical treatment and surgery groups.

Gedde SJ, ed. *Curbside Consultation in Glaucoma:*
49 Clinical Questions, Second Edition (pp 179–181)
© 2015 Taylor & Francis Group

Which Procedure Should I Choose?

Although the issue of when to perform surgery is a controversial one, even greater controversy exists regarding which type of surgery should be performed. In certain circumstances, filtering surgery is the best option, in others it may be a tube shunt, and still in others it may be cataract extraction with minimally invasive glaucoma surgery (MIGS). Each situation is unique, and the treatment plan should be tailored to the individual patient. Numerous studies can help guide our decision-making process.

In the first prospective, randomized trial of glaucoma drainage implants vs trabeculectomy, the Ahmed glaucoma valve and trabeculectomy for primary surgery were compared in 123 patients with an average follow-up of 31 months. The mean IOPs and adjunctive medications were comparable in the 2 groups. No statistically significant differences between groups were found for visual acuity, visual field, and short- or long-term complications. The cumulative probabilities of success were 68.1% for trabeculectomy and 69.8% for the Ahmed valve.[7,8]

The Tube Versus Trabeculectomy (TVT) Study was a multicenter clinical trial that compared the 350-mm[2] Baerveldt glaucoma implant to trabeculectomy with mitomycin-C in patients who had undergone previous cataract extraction with intraocular lens implantation and/or failed filtering surgery. The 5-year results showed that patients who underwent tube shunt surgery had a higher success rate than did the trabeculectomy group; cumulative probability of failure was 29.8% in the tube group and 46.9% in the trabeculectomy group. In terms of IOP reduction, there was no statistically significant difference between the tube shunt group and trabeculectomy group. Both procedures produced a significant reduction in pressure that was sustained at the 5-year follow-up, and there was a significant reduction in the use of supplemental medicines in both groups as well. Early postoperative complications were more frequently seen in the trabeculectomy group, although most were transient and self-limited. Late postoperative complications, reoperation for complications, differences in vision loss, and cataract extractions were not different between the 2 procedures. We can conclude from this study that trabeculectomy and tube shunt surgery will produce a similar reduction in IOP with a similar risk of serious complications in patient groups like those enrolled in the TVT Study.[9,10]

Situations exist where tube shunts may be preferred over trabeculectomy. Certain high-risk glaucomas such as neovascular glaucoma, uveitic glaucoma, iridocorneal endothelial syndrome, epithelial downgrowth, or aphakic glaucoma often do better with a glaucoma drainage device. Patients with a likely need for future surgery also do better with tube placement, as they are less prone to failure with subsequent ocular surgery relative to trabeculectomy. Finally, when compliance is an issue, tube shunts may be a better option, as their clinical course can be easier to manage and missed appointments do not jeopardize the success of surgery as much.

MIGS is a term that was coined by Ike Ahmed to refer to a number of glaucoma procedures that cause minimal trauma to the eye. MIGS are gaining popularity and should have a place in the glaucoma surgeon's armamentarium. Like any new procedure, there is a learning curve that must be overcome when these devices are first used. These procedures are best suited to treating mild to moderate glaucoma rather than those with more advanced disease, and they can often be combined with cataract surgery. Advantages of MIGS devices are that they often spare the conjunctiva, have a favorable safety profile, and allow for rapid recovery. Although the exact definition of what constitutes a minimally invasive glaucoma surgery will vary, the following devices are generally accepted to belong to the MIGS family: Trabectome (NeoMedix, Tustin, California), iStent (Glaukos, Laguna Hills, California), Xen Gel Stent (AqueSys, Irvine, California), Hydrus Intracanalicular Implant (Ivantis, Irvine, California), and the CyPass Micro-Stent (Transcend Medical, Menlo Park, California). Although many of these devices are still in US Food and Drug

Administration trials, there is hope that in the future, they will help bridge the gap between medical treatment and filtering surgery for patients with early disease.

For patients with moderate/advanced glaucoma, the best options are likely still a tube shunt or trabeculectomy. The data from the TVT Study suggest that the risk profile and IOP reduction are very similar between the 2 procedures, with neither surgery showing a clear superiority. I think it would be fair to say that when choosing between a trabeculectomy and tube shunt, the best option may ultimately be determined by the surgeon's level of comfort with each procedure.

References

1. Musch DC, Lichter PR, Guire KE, Standardi CL. The Collaborative Initial Glaucoma Treatment Study: study design, methods, and baseline characteristics of enrolled patients. *Ophthalmology.* 1999;106(4):653-662.
2. Lichter PR, Musch DC, Gillespie BW, et al. Interim clinical outcomes in the Collaborative Initial Glaucoma Treatment Study comparing initial treatment randomized to medications or surgery. *Ophthalmology.* 2001;108(11):1943 1953.
3. Musch DC, Gillespie BW, Lichter PR, Niziol LM, Janz NK. Visual field progression in the Collaborative Initial Glaucoma Treatment Study: the impact of treatment and other baseline factors. *Ophthalmology.* 2009;116(2):200-207.
4. Musch DC, Gillespie BW, Niziol LM, Lichter PR, Varma R. Intraocular pressure control and long-term visual field loss in the Collaborative Initial Glaucoma Treatment Study. *Ophthalmology.* 2011;118(9):1766-1773.
5. Migdal C, Gregory W, Hitchings R. Long-term functional outcome after early surgery compared with laser and medicine in open-angle glaucoma. *Ophthalmology.* 1994;101(10):1651-1657.
6. Hitchings RA, Migdal CS, Wormald R, Poinooswamy D, Fitzke F. The primary treatment trial: changes in the visual field analysis by computer-assisted perimetry. *Eye (Lond).* 1994;8(pt 1):117-120.
7. Wilson MR, Mendis U, Paliwal A, Haynatzka V. Long-term follow-up of primary glaucoma surgery with Ahmed glaucoma valve implant versus trabeculectomy. *Am J Ophthalmol.* 2003;136(3):464-470.
8. Wilson MR, Mendis U, Smith SD, Paliwal A. Ahmed glaucoma valve implant vs trabeculectomy in the surgical treatment of glaucoma: a randomized clinical trial. *Am J Ophthalmol.* 2000;130(3):267-273.
9. Gedde SJ, Schiffman JC, Feuer WJ, Herndon LW, Brandt JD, Budenz DL. Treatment outcomes in the Tube Versus Trabeculectomy (TVT) Study after five years of follow-up. *Am J Ophthalmol.* 2012;153(5):789-803.e782.
10. Gedde SJ, Herndon LW, Brandt JD, Budenz DL, Feuer WJ, Schiffman JC. Postoperative complications in the Tube Versus Trabeculectomy (TVT) Study during five years of follow-up. *Am J Ophthalmol.* 2012;153(5):804-814.e801.

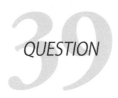

ARE ANTI-VASCULAR ENDOTHELIAL GROWTH FACTOR AGENTS USEFUL ADJUNCTS TO GLAUCOMA FILTERING SURGERY?

Rashmi G. Mathew, FRCOphth and
Keith Barton, MD, FRCP, FRCS

Although pharmacologic enhancement of trabeculectomy with either mitomycin-C (MMC) or 5-fluorouracil (5-FU) has significantly improved success rates, we have long felt that these agents are far from ideal. Their downfall, particularly MMC, is their nonspecific mechanism of action, which can result in thin-walled, avascular blebs that are prone to leakage, infection, and dysesthesia.

Episcleral fibrosis after trabeculectomy surgery occurs as a result of progressive fibroblast migration, proliferation, collagen deposition, and angiogenesis at the site of filtration surgery. An agent that specifically targets scar-forming fibroblasts would seem like the ideal prototype to improve trabeculectomy success rates without compromising bleb integrity. Furthermore, trabeculectomy surgery still lacks predictability in outcome, as the wound-healing response is variable. A cell-specific emissary may go some way toward improving predictability.

What Is the Evidence for Use of Vascular Endothelial Growth Factor Inhibitors, Such as Bevacizumab as Antifibrotic Agents, in Glaucoma Surgery?

Bevacizumab is a recombinant humanized monoclonal immunoglobulin (Ig) G1 antibody that binds to human vascular endothelial growth factor (VEGF) and inhibits its activity. It nonselectively inhibits all isoforms of VEGF. It is approved by the US Food and Drug Administration for the treatment of metastatic colorectal and breast cancer but is not licensed for ocular use.

Gedde SJ, ed. *Curbside Consultation in Glaucoma:
49 Clinical Questions, Second Edition* (pp 183–185)
© 2015 Taylor & Francis Group

As early as 1994, it was demonstrated that angiogenesis inhibitors had marked inhibitory effects on both Tenon fibroblast migration and proliferation, raising the possibility of a role for these agents in wound-healing modulation.[1]

Studies have shown that aqueous levels of VEGF in patients with primary open-angle glaucoma (POAG) undergoing cataract surgery or trabeculectomy surgery are significantly higher than those of patients without POAG.[2-4] Interestingly, 2 high-affinity VEGF tyrosine kinase receptors have been identified: fms-like tyrosine kinase 1 and kinase domain receptor, both of which are expressed on human Tenon fibroblasts.

Levels of VEGF have been shown to increase significantly after trabeculectomy surgery. Furthermore, in vitro studies show that the addition of VEGF stimulates fibroblast proliferation, and the addition of bevacizumab inhibits fibroblast proliferation in a dose-dependent manner.[4] At higher doses (more than 7.5 mg/mL), bevacizumab caused fibroblast death.[5]

Several animal studies have examined the effect of bevacizumab on bleb survival.[4,6,7] In the rabbit trabeculectomy model, bevacizumab has been shown to be superior to 5-FU, and there may be a synergistic effect when the 2 agents are used in combination.[7] Histologically, less scar tissue deposition has been found in the groups injected with subconjunctival bevacizumab.

Has Bevacizumab Shown Promising Results in the Clinical Setting?

The literature is awash with case series and small randomized studies using bevacizumab. The study methodology differs, and so direct comparisons are difficult. Some investigators have opted for combined use with MMC or 5-FU, while others have chosen no anti-metabolite. Most have chosen single injections,[8-12] and some have opted for multiple injections.[13,14] The route of administration also varies, with the majority choosing subconjunctival injections, but other authors have used intracameral injections[15,16] and 1 study chose intravitreal ranibizumab.[9]

The studies with no comparator arm have used either bevacizumab in isolation[8] or in conjunction with MMC.[10] The results appear favorable, although the follow-up periods are relatively short.

In those studies comparing bevacizumab with standard management of MMC or 5-FU, a single injection[11] of bevacizumab appears to fare worse than multiple injections[13] of bevacizumab. Of note, more absolute successes have been noted in the MMC/5-FU groups compared with the bevacizumab group, despite no overall difference in intraocular pressure between the groups.[11-13]

For those randomized to standard treatment with or without bevacizumab, the reports mostly suggest no difference in intraocular pressure between groups.[9,15,16] There does, however, seem to be a trend toward reduced postoperative interventions[16] (needlings and subconjunctival injections) in the bevacizumab groups, but this has not been confirmed in all studies. Another outcome measure that has been reported on is bleb morphology. Again, reports are mixed, with some authors seeing a trend toward avascularity[9,17] in bevacizumab groups and others reporting increased vascularity.[8,14]

Summary

The discovery of VEGF receptors on Tenon fibroblasts and the increased VEGF levels in patients with POAG, which elevate further after trabeculectomy surgery, point to a promising role for bevacizumab in both disrupting fibroblast proliferation and releasing VEGF into the aqueous and provide a strong argument for further investigating its role.

Lessons may be drawn from lerdelimumab, another monoclonal antibody, targeted against transforming growth factor β, which showed promising results in animal and human pilot trabeculectomy studies. Unfortunately, the randomized controlled clinical trial failed to achieve a statistically significant end point.[18] Questions remain in the investigators' minds whether a potentially useful clinical drug was lost due to suboptimal dosing or route of administration. It is therefore vital that the optimum route of administration and dosing frequency of bevacizumab are identified if its true potential in glaucoma filtration surgery is to be unlocked.

References

1. Wong J, Wang N, Miller JW, Schuman JS. Modulation of human fibroblast activity by selected angiogenesis inhibitors. *Exp Eye Res.* 1994;58:439-451.
2. Tripathi RC, Li J, Tripathi BJ, Chalam KV, Adamis AP. Increased level of vascular endothelial growth factor in aqueous humor of patients with neovascular glaucoma. *Ophthalmology.* 1998;105:232-237.
3. Hu DN, Ritch R, Liebmann J, Liu Y, Cheng B, Hu MS. Vascular endothelial growth factor is increased in aqueous humor of glaucomatous eyes. *J Glaucoma.* 2002;11:406-410.
4. Li Z, Van BT, V de Veire SI et al. Inhibition of vascular endothelial growth factor reduces scar formation after glaucoma filtration surgery. *Invest Ophthalmol Vis Sci.* 2009;50:5217-5225.
5. O'Neill EC, Qin Q, Van Bergen NJ et al. Antifibrotic activity of bevacizumab on human Tenon's fibroblasts in vitro. *Invest Ophthalmol Vis Sci.* 2010;51:6524-6532.
6. Memarzadeh F, Varma R, Lin LT et al. Postoperative use of bevacizumab as an antifibrotic agent in glaucoma filtration surgery in the rabbit. *Invest Ophthalmol Vis Sci.* 2009;50:3233-3237.
7. How A, Chua JL, Charlton A et al. Combined treatment with bevacizumab and 5-fluorouracil attenuates the postoperative scarring response after experimental glaucoma filtration surgery. *Invest Ophthalmol Vis Sci.* 2010;51:928-932.
8. Grewal DS, Jain R, Kumar H, Grewal SP. Evaluation of subconjunctival bevacizumab as an adjunct to trabeculectomy: a pilot study. *Ophthalmology.* 2008;115:2141-2145.
9. Kahook MY. Bleb morphology and vascularity after trabeculectomy with intravitreal ranibizumab: a pilot study. *Am J Ophthalmol.* 2010;150:399-403.
10. Biteli LG, Prata TS. Subconjunctival bevacizumab as an adjunct in first-time filtration surgery for patients with primary glaucomas. *Int Ophthalmol.* 2013;33:741-746.
11. Niloforushan N, Yadgari M, Kish SK, Nassiri N. Subconjunctival bevacizumab versus mitomycin C adjunctive to traveculectomy. *Am J Ophthalmol.* 2012;153:352-357.
12. Akkan JU, Cilsim S. Role of subconjunctival bevacizumab as an adjunctive to primary trabeculectomy: a prospective randomised comparative 1-year follow-up study. *J Glaucoma.* 2013 May 8. [Epub ahead of print]
13. Jurkowska-Dudzinska J, Kosior-Jarecka E, Zarnowski T. Comparison of the use of 5-fluorouracil and bevacizumab in primary trabeculectomy: results at 1 year. *Clin Experiment Ophthalmol.* 2012;40:e135-142.
14. Sengupta S, Venkatesh R, Ravindran RD. Safety and efficacy of using off-label bevacizumab versus mitomycin C to prevent bleb failure in a single-site phacotrabeculectomy by a randomized clinical trial. *J Glaucoma.* 2012;21:450-459.
15. Suh W, Kee C. The effect of bevacizumab on the outcome of trabeculectomy with 5-fluorouracil. *J Ocul Pharmacol Ther.* 2013;29:646-651.
16. Vandewalle E, Abegão Pinto L, Van Bergen T et al. Intracameral bevacizumab as an adjunct to trabeculectomy: a 1-year prospective, randomised study. *Br J Ophthalmol.* 2014;98:73-78.
17. Chua BE, Nguyen DQ, Qin Q et al. Bleb vascularity following post-trabeculectomy subconjunctival bevacizumab: a pilot study. *Clin Experiment Ophthalmol.* 2012;40:773-779.
18. CAT-152 0102 Trabeculectomy Study Group. A phase III study of subconjunctival human anti-transforming growth factor β2 monoclonal antibody (CAT–152) to prevent scarring after first-time trabeculectomy. *Ophthalmology.* 2007;114:1822-1830.

Further Reading

Mathew R, Barton K. Anti-vascular endothelial growth factor therapy in glaucoma filtration surgery. *Am J Ophthalmol* 2011;152:10-15.

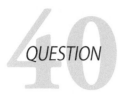
WHAT ARE SURGICAL PEARLS FOR PERFORMING TRABECULECTOMY?

Ronald L. Fellman, MD and
Davinder S. Grover, MD, MPH

Glaucoma surgeons have the opportunity to improve flow into the patient's natural drainage system through a canal-based procedure or create a new drainage system through limbal transcleral filtration or drainage implants. Trabeculectomy, a type of guarded filtration, lowers intraocular pressure (IOP) by rerouting the flow of aqueous from a dysfunctional outflow system to the subconjunctival space, producing a bleb. The potential problems associated with external filtration include hypotony, reduced acuity, scarring, leaks, bleb dysesthesia, blebitis, and endophthalmitis. These risks are considerable but are warranted in patients who require a significant drop in IOP to change the course of their disease. A recent large study found target IOP was achieved at 4 years in 70% of filtered eyes, with 15% of eyes requiring further glaucoma surgery and 9% requiring surgery for bleb-related problems.[1]

The need for filtration surgery has decreased in patients with glaucoma who have mild to moderate disease and tolerate topical therapy because of the relative success of microinvasive canal-based surgery, especially in conjunction with cataract surgery.

One of the difficulties associated with trabeculectomy is the many intraoperative and postoperative clinical decisions that are necessary to achieve meaningful filtration through a scleral flap, with just the right amount of flow to create a long-lasting asymptomatic diffuse, pale but not avascular bleb. This chapter reviews the critical steps to achieve this goal.

Gedde SJ, ed. *Curbside Consultation in Glaucoma:*
49 Clinical Questions, Second Edition (pp 187–192)
© 2015 Taylor & Francis Group

Figure 40-1. Proper exposure, peritomy, and management of Tenon's capsule. (A) The corneal traction suture provides excellent exposure of the operative site. The peritomy starts with a radial wing incision, which provides good exposure for creation of the scleral flap. The incision is continued along the limbus. The sharp Westcott scissors straddle the insertion site of both Tenon's capsule (white arrow) and the conjunctiva (black arrow). (B) Dissect far posteriorly underneath both conjunctiva and Tenon's capsule (black arrow) to create an adequate space for diffuse filtration.

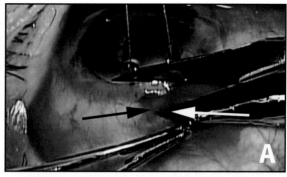

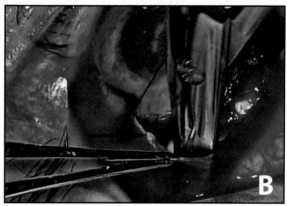

Exposure, Conjunctival Peritomy, and Management of Tenon's Capsule

A traction suture is vital for optimal exposure in both fornix- and limbus-based approaches. Failure to obtain adequate exposure of the operative site is the most common first misstep of filtration surgery. Inadequate exposure during a limbus-based approach can lead to an anteriorly displaced conjunctival incision, which is a risk factor for symptomatic, pale avascular blebs that tend to leak. This simple misstep can lead to a lifetime of ocular misery due to bleb dysesthesia.

The authors prefer a fornix-based trabeculectomy (the focus of this chapter) because of more favorable long-term bleb characteristics, and if future glaucoma surgery is necessary, the conjunctival dissection is safer and simpler. A large retrospective study found no statistically significant difference in IOP control between limbus- and fornix-based trabeculectomies, but limbus-based filters were higher and more avascular and slightly more prone to blebitis.[2]

The peritomy may be constructed directly at the limbus or slightly posterior to allow a short skirt of conjunctiva to help with wound closure. With either approach, the anterior limbal attachment of Tenon's capsule should be incorporated into the peritomy to facilitate the combined posterior dissection of Tenon's capsule and conjunctiva (Figure 40-1).

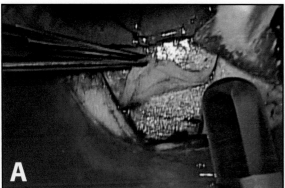

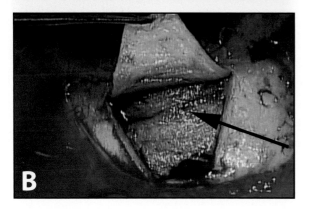

Figure 40-2. Dissection of the scleral flap. (A) The flap is constructed with a crescent blade and .12 toothed forceps. It should be a uniform two-thirds thickness flap, dissected into clear cornea. (B) The arrow denotes the location of the scleral spur. This is the posterior extent of the proposed sclerostomy site; otherwise, the scleral spur may be unroofed, creating an unwanted cyclodialysis cleft.

Antimetabolite Decision

Most surgeons employ mitomycin-C (MMC) to inhibit fibrosis at the filtration area. There is still controversy over the concentration and duration of application (even between the authors), but in general, the authors prefer a broad application of either MMC 0.2 mg/cc or 0.4 mg/cc for 2 to 4 minutes with the sponges placed well posteriorly and not directly over the scleral flap.

Fashion Scleral Flap, Preplace Sutures, and Paracentesis

There are a variety of shapes and methods to create the scleral flap. The authors typically create a two-thirds thickness trapezoidal-shaped uniform flap that extends into clear cornea to allow adequate room and coverage for the sclerostomy. Flaps are much more difficult in highly myopic eyes with thin sclera or eyes with prior limbal surgery (Figure 40-2). Under this circumstance, the scleral flap may be created with an angled crescent blade by forming a scleral tunnel and opening the edges.

Figure 40-3. Preparation of the sclerostomy site. (A) After preplaced sutures and a temporal paracentesis, a super sharp blade is used to enter the anterior chamber at the anterior extent of the sclerostomy site, parallel to the iris. Use a Kelly punch to remove the corneoscleral tissue to create the sclerostomy site. (B) Proper appearance of a well-prepared sclerostomy site with adequate size, scleral flap coverage, location, and peripheral iridectomy.

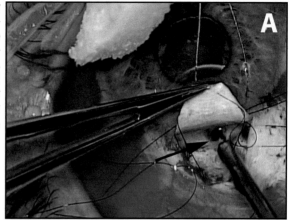

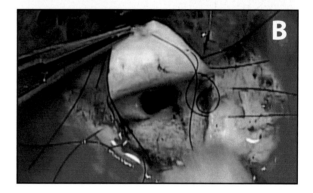

Sclerostomy Site and Conjunctival Closure

Wound construction in and around the sclerostomy site is critical to a successful outcome. One must avoid excessive early flow through the filter, which may lead to suprachoroidal events.[3] Although there are a variety of methods to create the sclerostomy, the authors prefer a Kelly (or similar type) punch to remove the limbal tissue. The opening should be large enough to prevent early closure but with adequate enough boundaries to allow scleral flap coverage. It is important to achieve intraoperative flow through the filter. A peripheral iridectomy is still recommended in most cases to prevent obstruction of the opening by the iris and especially in eyes prone to inflammation from uveitis or diabetes (Figure 40-3). The scleral flap is closed with 3 to 5 interrupted 10-0 nylon sutures in a manner that allows slow aqueous egress from around the flap while maintaining a physiologic pressure and a deep anterior chamber. A watertight conjunctival closure is imperative to promote early bleb formation. The authors are firm believers that incorporation of Tenon's capsule into the conjunctival closure aids in preventing early wound leaks and is helpful in the long term to prevent bleb dysesthesia and blebitis (Figure 40-4). There are a variety of successful conjunctival closures, including the described conjunctivopexy mattress suture technique. Most of the suture techniques incorporate a component of the Wise technique, a horizontal mattress variant.[4] Review a book chapter to learn more about filtration surgery and the intricacies of wound closure.[5] At the completion of the case, 8 to 12 mg of triamcinolone acetonide can be injected into the inferior fornix to suppress scarring.

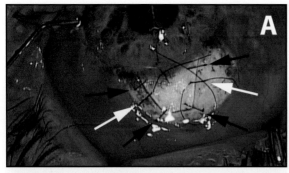

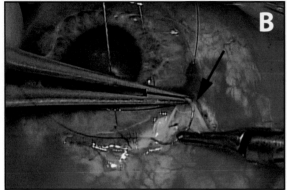

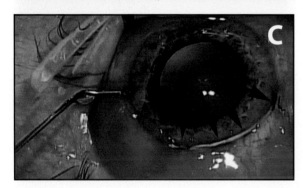

Figure 40-4. Closure of the sclerostomy site and conjunctiva. (A) The 4 main sutures (black arrows) are closed and fluid instilled into the anterior chamber to judge the flow through the flap. The middle sutures (white arrows) are adjusted to allow flow through the filter to prevent a pressure spike on postoperative day 1. Considerable time is spent judging flow and adjusting wound architecture to achieve reasonable intraoperative flow through the scleral flap. (B) The radial wing is closed first with a tapered 9-0 nylon needle (Ethicon 2829; Ethicon, Somerville, New Jersey) while incorporating Tenon's capsule (black arrow). (C) Tenon's capsule is captured underneath the conjunctiva and incorporated into the conjunctival closure (black arrows). Several interrupted 9-0 nylon sutures (2890 Ethicon) are used to close the limbal peritomy. This is a variant of the Wise technique; a horizontal mattress suture tacks the tissue down at the suture point and tethers the tissue between bites to prevent leaks.

The intraoperative and postoperative management of filtration surgery remains an art, as exemplified by the techniques outlined. It is prudent to test the wound margin for leaks in the early postoperative period no matter the circumstances. Consider mydriatic cycloplegics to stabilize the blood aqueous barrier and prevent spasm of the ciliary body with subsequent eye pain and likely reduced aqueous production. An injected bleb signifies potential failure requiring either increased flow through the flap and/or typically a boost of topical corticosteroid. Strive for the perfect bleb that is pale but not avascular, low but not flat, and diffuse but not extending into the palpebral fissure (Figure 40-5). The perfect bleb is an art, not a science.

Figure 40-5. Bleb outcome morphology. (A) This bleb is a thin, avascular, undesirable dysesthetic bleb. This type of bleb is bothersome and has intermittent leaks. A very uncomfortable and worrisome situation. (B) This bleb is pale but not avascular with a few vessels on the conjunctiva. It is diffuse and does not leak. This patient is asymptomatic with no history of a leak and maintains an IOP of 12 mm Hg without topical therapy.

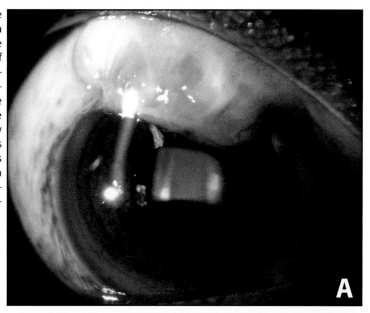

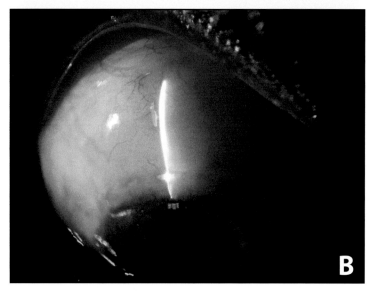

References

1. Jampel HD, Solus JF, Tracey PA, et al. Outcomes and bleb-related complications of trabeculectomy. *Ophthalmology*. 2012;19:712-722.

2. Solus JF, Jampel HD, Tracey PA, et al. Comparison of limbus-based and fornix-based trabeculectomy: success, bleb-related complication, and bleb morphology. *Ophthalmology*. 2012;119:703-711.

3. Fellman RL. Choroidal effusion and hemorrhage. In: Feldman RM, Bell NP, eds. *Complications of Glaucoma Surgery*. Oxford, UK: Oxford University Press; 2013.

4. Wise JB. Mitomycin-compatible suture technique for fornix-based conjunctival flaps in glaucoma filtration surgery. *Arch Ophthalmol*. 1993;111:992-997.

5. Fellman RL, Grover DS. Trabeculectomy, Chapter 77. In: Shaarawy TM, Sherwood MB, Hitchings RA, Crowston JG, eds. *Glaucoma: Surgical Management*, vol 2. 2nd edition. London, UK: Elsevier Limited 2015.

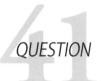

WHAT ARE PEARLS FOR THE POSTOPERATIVE MANAGEMENT OF TRABECULECTOMY AND ITS ASSOCIATED COMPLICATIONS?

Ahmad A. Aref, MD

Although surgeon skill and technique are undoubtedly important components of trabeculectomy surgical outcome, one may argue that postoperative management strategies determine ultimate surgical success.

The timing of episcleral fibrosis under the trabeculectomy flap is individually variable. Therefore, frequent postoperative follow-up visits are necessary to allow for appropriate adjustment of medications and timing of postoperative maneuvers in each patient. I prefer to see patients the first day after surgery or even the day of surgery if the patient is functionally monocular or deemed to be at high risk for postoperative complications. Patients are followed every few days thereafter throughout the immediate postoperative period. Topical corticosteroids are administered at least 4 times daily to help prevent excessive episcleral fibrosis, with tapering based on conjunctival vascularity. More recently available topical corticosteroid formulations such as difluprednate (Durezol; Alcon Laboratories, Fort Worth, Texas) require less frequent dosing due to enhanced potency. Although evidence is limited to support the administration of a topical antibiotic, these agents are often administered for the first postoperative week. Topical cycloplegics are helpful in deepening the anterior chamber, especially in phakic individuals.

Intraoperatively, the surgeon may aim for an immediate postoperative intraocular pressure (IOP) slightly higher than target to decrease the risk of hypotony-related complications. This necessitates a strategy for increasing aqueous flow in the postoperative period. When an adjunctive antifibrotic agent such as mitomycin-C or 5-fluorouracil has been used, I prefer to wait at least 2 to 3 weeks before attempting to increase aqueous flow to allow sufficient time for early healing and to decrease the risk of hypotony-related complications. Trabeculectomy flow may be increased by mechanical pressure adjacent to the scleral flap (Carlo-Traverso maneuver), laser suture-lysis, or removal of a releasable suture. The Carlo-Traverso maneuver typically only provides transient IOP lowering. Laser suture-lysis offers longer term flow enhancement but requires adequate

Gedde SJ, ed. *Curbside Consultation in Glaucoma:*
49 Clinical Questions, Second Edition (pp 193–196)
© 2015 Taylor & Francis Group

Figure 41-1. Intraoperative view of a circumferential compression suture placed across the scleral flap to decrease aqueous flow due to bleb hyperfiltration. This technique was described by Suner, et al.[4]

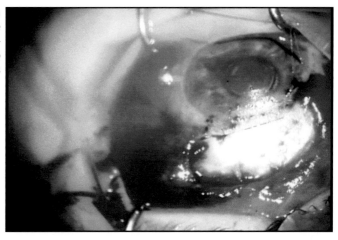

subconjunctival visualization. Releasable suture removal is also an effective strategy, but sutures sometimes break upon attempted removal. When episcleral fibrosis renders the aforementioned maneuvers ineffective, bleb revision surgery may be indicated to lower IOP to a target range. My preference is to combine bleb revision surgery or "needling" with reapplication of an antifibrotic agent to inhibit further episcleral scarring.

The importance of early recognition of postoperative complications cannot be overstated. In the Tube Versus Trabeculectomy Study, most early postoperative complications were transient in nature with minimal effect on final outcome when managed appropriately.[1] Early hypotony-related complications may be due to aqueous hyposecretion, overfiltration, or conjunctival wound leakage. Patients experiencing postoperative hypotony should avoid any activities that may cause ocular strain and increase the risk of a suprachoroidal hemorrhage. Testing of conjunctival wound integrity should be performed with a fluorescein strip on every visit within the postoperative period. A confirmed leak may be initially treated with a bandage contact lens and/or aqueous suppression. Persistence of the leak beyond a few weeks requires surgical revision in either a minor procedure room or the operating room.

Overfiltration may be transient and treated conservatively as physiologic episcleral healing occurs; however, revision surgery (Figure 41-1) is sometimes necessary to treat persistent related complications. Anterior chamber shallowing may result in corneal decompensation and/or cataract progression. In this scenario, a topical cycloplegic may deepen the anterior chamber. Lenticulo-corneal (as opposed to irido-corneal) "touch" requires prompt intervention. I prefer to initially re-form the anterior chamber with a cohesive viscoelastic device while addressing the underlying cause of hypotony. Younger, myopic individuals are at greater risk for hypotony maculopathy. It is important to obtain digital imaging (Figure 41-2) in suspected cases as clinical signs are often subtle.[2] Vertical sections should be obtained as macular folds may be missed if only horizontal scans are obtained. Macular folds associated with hypotony tend to be oriented along the 180-degree meridian and may not be detected if the imaging sections are aligned along the axis of the chorioretinal folds. Treatment should be directed at the underlying cause of hypotony. Choroidal effusions are often transient in nature and may be closely observed. However, "kissing" choroidals usually require surgical drainage to decrease risk of secondary adverse retinal events. Postoperative peripheral suprachoroidal hemorrhages may also be initially observed but often take longer to spontaneously resolve. Larger suprachoroidal hemorrhages associated with apposition, uncontrolled IOP, lenticulo-corneal touch, and/or intractable pain require prompt surgical drainage.

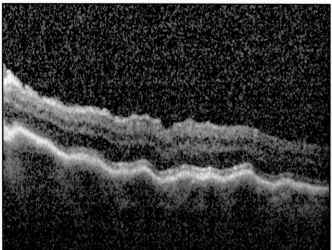

Figure 41-2. Optical coherence tomography scan image of hypotony maculopathy after trabeculectomy surgery. Clinical funduscopic examination appeared to be unremarkable.

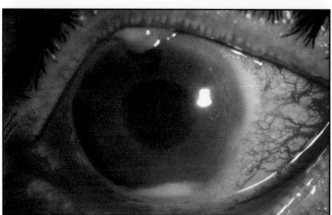

Figure 41-3. Late-onset bleb-related endophthalmitis occurring several years after the original operation. (Reprinted with permission of Dr. Steven J. Gedde.)

Endophthalmitis may occur in either the early or the late (Figure 41-3) postoperative periods. Any patient who has undergone trabeculectomy surgery must be educated with regard to the symptoms of this process with clear instructions to immediately call his or her local eye care provider should they occur. Individuals with narrow anterior chamber angles are at risk for postoperative aqueous misdirection. This process should be strongly considered in the differential diagnosis of patients presenting with postoperative elevation in IOP and flat anterior chamber in the setting of a patent iridectomy and unremarkable funduscopic examination. In pseudophakic individuals, Nd:YAG laser capsulotomy/hyaloidotomy along with cycloplegia may break the attack, but pars plana vitrectomy, hyaloido-zonulectomy, and iridectomy may ultimately be required.[3]

Trabeculectomy surgery requires an intensive postoperative management protocol by patients and surgeons alike. Potential complications may be vision threatening. Attention to detail, prompt management strategies, and proper patient education are keys to success.

References

1. Gedde SJ, Herndon LW, Brandt JD, et al. Postoperative complications in the Tube Versus Trabeculectomy (TVT) Study during five years of follow-up. *Am J Ophthalmol.* 2012;153:804-814.
2. Budenz DL, Schwartz K, Gedde SJ. Occult hypotony maculopathy diagnosed with optical coherence tomography. *Arch Ophthalmol.* 2005;123:113-114.
3. Bitrian E, Caprioli J. Pars plana anterior vitrectomy, hyaloido-zonulectomy, and iridectomy for aqueous humor misdirection. *Am J Ophthalmol.* 2010;150:82-87.
4. Suner IJ, Greenfield DS, Miller MP, et al. Hypotony maculopathy after filtering surgery mitomycin C. Incidence and treatment. *Ophthalmology.* 1997;104:207-214.

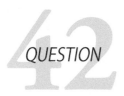

WHAT ARE SURGICAL PEARLS FOR PERFORMING AQUEOUS SHUNT IMPLANTATION?

Steven J. Gedde, MD

Several different aqueous shunts (or glaucoma drainage implants) are commercially available, and they all share a common design consisting of a silicone tube that connects to an end plate. Shunts differ with respect to the size, shape, and material composition of the end plate.[1] These devices may be classified as valved or nonvalved implants, depending on whether a valve mechanism is present to limit flow through the tube if the intraocular pressure (IOP) becomes too low.

The surgical technique for implanting aqueous shunts is similar, irrespective of the type of implant used. A careful ocular examination should be performed preoperatively to plan the surgical approach, and meticulous surgical technique serves to minimize intraoperative and postoperative complications. The procedure is usually performed under local anesthesia with a retrobulbar or peribulbar block.

Conjunctival Incision

The superotemporal quadrant is generally selected as the site for placement of single-plate implants because surgical exposure is better and postoperative strabismus is less frequent. The superonasal quadrant should be avoided due to the increased risk of producing motility disturbances.[2] A limbus-based or fornix-based conjunctival flap is dissected, depending on the surgeon's preference. No significant differences in surgical outcomes were observed with limbus- and fornix-based flaps in a retrospective study of aqueous shunts.[3] I prefer a fornix-based flap because it optimizes surgical exposure for attachment of the end plate and insertion of the tube (Figure 42-1). Double-plate devices require a 180-degree incision, while single-plate implants may be inserted through a 90- to 100-degree incision. A relaxing incision on either side of the peritomy will improve exposure.

Gedde SJ, ed. *Curbside Consultation in Glaucoma:*
49 Clinical Questions, Second Edition (pp 197–201)
© 2015 Taylor & Francis Group

Figure 42-1. A fornix-based conjunctival flap is dissected.

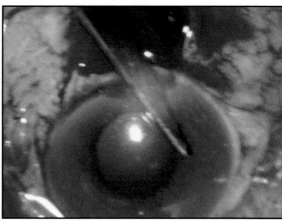

Quadrant Dissection

The conjunctiva and Tenon's capsule are dissected from the sclera to create space for the implant. A traction suture placed in the peripheral cornea may be used to enhance exposure, and this same suture may be incorporated into the closure of a fornix-based conjunctival flap. Cautery is applied to bleeding episcleral vessels.

Attachment of the End Plate

The implant is placed in antibiotic solution before insertion. Adjacent rectus muscles are identified with muscle hooks, and the end plate is positioned between the muscles. The lateral wings of the Baerveldt glaucoma implant were designed for positioning under the rectus muscles. I use a caliper to ensure that the end plate is attached to sclera at a measured distance of 10 mm posterior to the limbus. I think this is particularly important when using the Baerveldt implant, as it prevents crowding of the muscle insertions by the plate and may help reduce the chance of postoperative diplopia. A nonabsorbable suture (I prefer 8-0 nylon) is used to attach the end plate, and the knots are rotated into the fixation holes of the implant to prevent erosion through the conjunctiva (Figure 42-2). When using double-plate implants, one plate is positioned in each of two quadrants and the tube connecting them may be positioned under or over the rectus muscle.

Preparation of the Implant

PRIMING VALVED IMPLANTS

Valved implants must be "primed" by injecting balanced salt solution (BSS) through the tube using a cannula. This serves to break the surface tension between the 2 silicone sheets of the Ahmed implant, so the valve mechanism can function. Irrigating with BSS confirms that the valve slits in the Krupin implant allow flow.

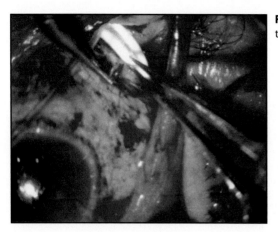

Figure 42-2. The end plate is sutured to sclera through the fixation holes of the implant.

RESTRICTION OF AQUEOUS FLOW IN NONVALVED IMPLANTS

Nonvalved implants require a restriction of aqueous flow until encapsulation of the end plate occurs. This is necessary to avoid overfiltration in the early postoperative period and to minimize the risk of hypotony. A 2-stage implantation technique may be employed in which the end plate is attached to sclera in the first stage of the procedure, and the tube is later inserted into the anterior chamber after 4 to 8 weeks in the second stage. Single-stage implantation is more commonly performed with temporary tube ligation using a polyglactin or prolene suture, or tube obstruction with a luminal suture. I generally ligate the tube with a 7-0 polyglactin suture near the tube-plate junction, and a watertight closure is confirmed by attempting to irrigate BSS through the tube. The polyglactin suture reliably lyses 4 to 6 weeks postoperatively, causing spontaneous opening of the tube.

Temporary flow restriction makes nonvalved implants nonfunctional immediately following surgery. Tube fenestration is an effective way of providing IOP reduction in the early postoperative period.[4] I prefer to fenestrate with a TG-140 or TG-160 needle (Ethicon, Somerville, New Jersey) just anterior to the polyglactin ligature, and 1 to 3 fenestrations are placed along the tube depending on the preoperative IOP level.

Insertion of the Tube

The tube is draped across the cornea and cut with an anterior bevel so a 2- to 3-mm segment of tube extends into the anterior chamber from the site of limbal entry. A 23-gauge needle is used to make a track for the tube, beginning 3 mm posterior to the limbus and tunneling through sclera to allow entry into the anterior chamber just above the iris plane (Figure 42-3). This size needle creates a tight entry wound for the tube, reducing leakage around the tube. The tube is inserted through the needle track with tying forceps or a tube insertion forceps. Proper positioning of the tube away from the corneal endothelium should be confirmed. Alternatively, the tube may be inserted through the pars plana in an eye that has had a complete pars plana vitrectomy or into the ciliary sulcus with the tube beveled posteriorly in an eye with a posterior chamber intraocular lens implant.

Figure 42-3. A 23-gauge needle is used to make an entry incision into the anterior chamber.

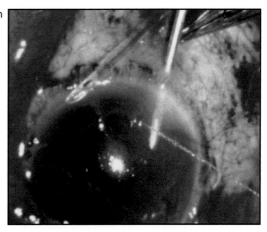

Figure 42-4. The limbal portion of the tube is covered with a scleral patch graft.

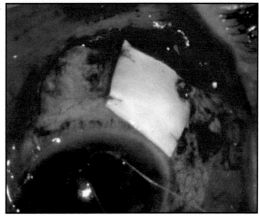

Tube Coverage With a Patch Graft

The limbal portion of the tube is covered with a patch graft measuring approximately 4 × 4 mm (Figure 42-4). Cornea, sclera, pericardium, fascia lata, or dura mater are all acceptable patch graft materials. I favor donor cornea split to half thickness because of its superior cosmetic appearance, especially with inferiorly positioned implants. Various techniques have also been described for tube insertion through a scleral tunnel without a donor patch graft.

Conjunctival Closure

The conjunctiva is closed by reapproximating it to the limbus with mattress sutures when using a fornix-based flap or using a running closure for limbus-based flaps and radial relaxing incisions.

References

1. Gedde SJ, Panarelli JF, Banitt MR, Lee RK. Evidence-based comparison of aqueous shunts. *Curr Opin Ophthalmol.* 2013;24:87-95.

2. Christmann LM, Wilson ME. Motility disturbances after Molteno implants. *J Pediatr Ophthalmol Strabismus.* 1992;29:44-48.
3. Suhr AW, Lim MC, Trandt JD, Izquierdo JC, Willits N. Outcomes of fornix-based versus limbus-based conjunctival incisions for glaucoma drainage device implant. *J Glaucoma.* 2012;21:523-529.
4. Emerick GT, Gedde SJ, Budnez DL. Tube fenestrations in Baerveldt glaucoma implant surgery: 1-year results compared with standard implant surgery. *J Glaucoma.* 2002;11:340-346.

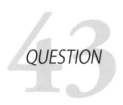

What Are Pearls for Postoperative Management of Aqueous Shunt Implantation and Its Associated Complications?

Joseph F. Panarelli, MD and
Paul A. Sidoti, MD

Aqueous shunts are being used with increasing frequency as an alternative to trabeculectomy. Aqueous shunt implantation is associated with similar postoperative complications as occurs with standard filtering surgery. In addition, unique complications may develop related to implantation of a device. Careful surgical technique and postoperative care can minimize the risk of complications and optimize outcomes.

Postoperative Care

Following aqueous shunt surgery, patients are evaluated on the first postoperative day and started on topical antibiotic and corticosteroid drops. If the intraocular pressure (IOP) is elevated, prior glaucoma medications can be resumed. Patients then follow up at 1 week and every 1 to 2 weeks thereafter until a stable level of IOP is observed. Corticosteroid drops can be reduced during the early postoperative period. However, an increase in topical corticosteroid therapy is generally required when a nonvalved implant opens, as this event is usually associated with increased inflammation. Once the inflammation is controlled, the corticosteroid medication can be gradually tapered over a few weeks.

Gedde SJ, ed. *Curbside Consultation in Glaucoma:*
49 Clinical Questions, Second Edition (pp 203–206)
© 2015 Taylor & Francis Group

Postoperative Complications

Early recognition and appropriate treatment of postoperative complications is important in ensuring the best surgical result after aqueous shunt implantation. We discuss some of the more common complications seen with aqueous shunt surgery.

MOTILITY DISTURBANCES

The incidence of diplopia has been reported to range from 1.4% to 37%, and persistent postoperative strabismus has ranged from 2.1% to 77% in case series of tube shunts.[1] Restrictive strabismus may occur because of scarring between the rectus or oblique muscles and the implant[2] or due to a crowding effect from a large bleb with limitation of extraocular motility.[3] Motility disturbances were investigated prospectively in the Tube Versus Trabeculectomy (TVT) Study, and the rate of persistent diplopia was 6%.[1]

Diplopia can be transient and often resolves within the first 6 months after surgery. If it persists, prisms can sometimes correct small deviations, and aqueous suppressants may prove helpful for symptomatic diplopia related to a large-sized bleb. However, there are times when patients ultimately need strabismus surgery for correction or, rarely, removal of the implant. To help minimize the risk of postoperative strabismus, surgeons should ensure that the implant is placed at least 9 to 10 mm posterior to the limbus, behind the rectus muscle insertions. The wings of larger implants should be placed completely beneath the proper muscles. When working in the superotemporal quadrant, particular care should be taken to avoid placement beneath the superior oblique muscle. We avoid superonasal placement of tube shunts because it has been described as a risk factor for motility disturbances postoperatively.[2]

TUBE/PLATE EROSION

A meta-analysis was recently performed of 38 prior studies that included 3255 eyes of 3105 patients who underwent tube shunt implantation.[4] The overall incidence of tube exposure was 2.0% with an average rate of exposure of 0.09% per month. No difference in the frequency of exposure was observed among the Ahmed, Baerveldt, and Molteno implants in this study. Tube erosion usually develops a few millimeters behind the limbus and may relate to focal elevation created at this location when the tube changes direction to enter the eye combined with exposure and repetitive trauma from eyelid movement.

We always cover the limbal portion of the tube with a patch graft to minimize the risk of tube erosion. Cornea, sclera, pericardium, fascia lata, and dura mater are all acceptable patch graft materials. Alternatively, various techniques have been described for tube insertion through a scleral tunnel without a donor patch graft.[5,6] If tube erosion is detected, prompt surgical repair is indicated. An exposed tube provides a potential route by which bacteria can gain access to the eye and is a known risk factor for endophthalmitis.[7] Direct closure of the conjunctiva over the area of tube exposure is generally inadequate to resolve the problem, and a new patch graft should be placed under a conjunctival flap. We believe that exposure of a tube shunt plate is best managed by removal of the implant and placement of a new implant in a different quadrant. In our experience, plate erosions frequently recur despite attempts at surgical repair.

CORNEAL EDEMA

One of the most concerning complications of tube shunt surgery is corneal edema. Although it is preferable to place the tube safely away from the cornea, this is not always possible, especially when the anterior chamber is shallow and/or peripheral anterior synechiae are present. Numerous mechanisms have been postulated for corneal failure in patients with a tube shunt in the anterior chamber. Constant direct contact between the tube and endothelium will rapidly lead to endothelial cell loss and often produces focal corneal edema. Intermittent contact can occur during eye rubbing and squeezing if a tube is positioned too anteriorly, particularly if the IOP is low. Intraoperative and postoperative alterations in aqueous flow and a breakdown in the blood/aqueous barrier can also potentially lead to further endothelial compromise.

We much prefer to have a tube touching the iris than the cornea, and we have not encountered problems with chronic iritis with tube-iris contact. Anterior positioning of the tube with constant or intermittent corneal contact, progressive decline in the corneal endothelial cell count, or localized corneal edema in the region of the tube is best treated with repositioning of the tube to a more posterior location. If there is inadequate space in the anterior chamber, the tube may be positioned in the ciliary sulcus or pars plana. A complete pars plana vitrectomy with trimming of the vitreous base at the site of tube insertion is required for pars plana tube placement. Progressive endothelial cell loss may necessitate a penetrating keratoplasty or Descemet's stripping automated endothelial keratoplasty (DSAEK), and consideration should be given to repositioning the tube at the time of corneal transplantation.

HYPOTONY-RELATED COMPLICATIONS

Hypotony may develop after tube shunt surgery, along with associated complications, including choroidal effusions, anterior chamber shallowing, corneal edema, hypotony maculopathy, cystoid macular edema, and suprachoroidal hemorrhage. Valved implants have been reported to have a lower risk of hypotony-related complications compared with nonvalved implants,[8] and valved devices seem especially desirable in situations in which aqueous hyposecretion may be present (eg, uveitic glaucoma, prior cyclodestruction). However, early postoperative hypotony may still develop with valved implants due to inadequate valve function, and we routinely inject Healon into the anterior chamber at the conclusion of these cases in the operating room. Hypotony after nonvalved tube shunt placement generally occurs following release of a tube ligature, and we will often fill the anterior chamber with Healon immediately after laser suture lysis in the office.

BLEB ENCAPSULATION

Failure to control IOP after tube shunt surgery may occur secondary to excessive thickening of the fibrous capsule around the end plate. This complication is analogous to an encapsulated bleb that develops after trabeculectomy, and it is generally treated in a similar fashion with glaucoma medications. Some surgeons have suggested that bleb encapsulation is less likely to develop if the IOP is maintained in the low teens postoperatively. As a result, we have become more aggressive in restarting glaucoma medications soon after tube ligature release or following the development of a capsule with a flow-restricting device. The hypertensive bleb phase frequently resolves over the course of several weeks to months. A higher rate of bleb capsule thickening has been observed with valved than with nonvalved implants.[9-11] Immediate filtration of aqueous rich in inflammatory mediators may stimulate the creation of a thicker capsule following valved implant placement, and delayed aqueous flow with nonvalved implants may elicit a lesser fibrotic reaction.

Summary

Careful preoperative planning and proper surgical technique can help reduce the aforementioned complications and ensure the best possible outcome for your patient. When complications do arise, early recognition and appropriate treatment are key to optimizing long-term surgical success.

References

1. Gedde SJ, Herndon LW, Brandt JD, Budenz DL, Feuer WJ, Schiffman JC; Tube Versus Trabeculectomy Group. Postoperative complications in the Tube Versus Trabeculectomy (TVT) Study during five years of follow-up. *Am J Ophthalmol.* 2012;153(5):804-814.
2. Christmann LM, Wilson ME. Motility disturbances after Molteno implants. *J Pediatr Ophthalmol Strabismus.* 1992;29:44-48.
3. Ball SF, Ellis GS, Herrington RC, Liang K. Brown's superior oblique tendon syndrome after Baerveldt glaucoma implant. *Arch Ophthalmol.* 1992;110:1368.
4. Stewart WC, Kristoffersen CJ, Demos CM, et al. Incidence of conjunctival exposure following drainage device implantation in patients with glaucoma. *Eur J Ophthalmol.* 2010;20:124-130.
5. Ollila M, Falk Q, Airaksinen PJ. Placing the Molteno implant in a long scleral tunnel to prevent postoperative tube exposure. *Acta Ophthalmol Scand.* 2005;83:302-305.
6. Rossiter-thornton L, Azar D, Leong J, et al. Graft-free Molteno tube insertion: 10 year outcomes. *Br J Ophthalmol.* 2010;94:665-666.
7. Gedde SJ, Scott IS, Tabandeh H, et al. Late endophthalmitis associated with glaucoma drainage implants. *Ophthalmology.* 2001;108:1323-1327.
8. Tsai JC, Johnson CC, Kammer JA, Dietrich MS. The Ahmed shunt versus the Baerveldt shunt for refractory glaucoma, II: longer-term outcomes from a single surgeon. *Ophthalmology.* 2006;113:913-917.
9. Tsai JC, Johnson CC, Dietrich MS. The Ahmed shunt versus the Baerveldt shunt for refractory glaucoma: a single-surgeon comparison of outcome. *Ophthalmology.* 2003;11:1814-1821.
10. Ayyala RS, Zurakowski D, Monshizadeh R, et al. Comparison of double-plate Molteno and Ahmed glaucoma valve in patients with advanced uncontrolled glaucoma. *Ophthalmic Surg Lasers.* 2002;33:94-101.
11. Nassiri N, Kamali G, Rahnavardi M, et al. Ahmed glaucoma valve and single-plate Molteno implants in treatment of refractory glaucoma: a comparative study. *Am J Ophthalmol.* 2010;149:893-902.

WHICH AQUEOUS SHUNT SHOULD I USE?

Donald L. Budenz, MD, MPH

With the increasing use of aqueous shunts in the management of glaucoma, I am often asked, "Which aqueous shunt should I use?" This is not a simple question to answer, but there is some help from the peer review literature and anecdotal experience that may help guide us. A recent outstanding in-depth review of this topic is also available.[1]

Aqueous shunts differ in terms of material, size of the end plate, and whether they are valved or nonvalved. All of these factors enter into the decision-making process of which to choose for an individual patient. In addition, different diagnoses and patient factors should also be considered. Aqueous shunt surgery should not be a "one-size-fits-all" process.

The 3 most commonly used aqueous shunts are the Ahmed Glaucoma Valve (New World Medical, Rancho Cucamonga, California), Baerveldt Glaucoma Implant (Abbott Medical Optics, Santa Ana, California), and the Molteno Implant (IOP Ophthalmics, Costa Mesa, California). Most of the current models of these implants are made of silicone rather than polypropylene, as silicone may result in less postoperative inflammation, which presumably results in less scarring and increased success. While the tubes themselves are identical in the 3 implants, their end plates are dramatically different. The Ahmed implant has a valved end plate that is 96 mm^2 (model FP8), 184 mm^2 (model FP7), or 191 mm^2 (model M4). The Baerveldt implant has a nonvalved end plate that is either 250 mm^2 (model 103-250) or 350 mm^2 (model 101-350), and the Molteno 3 implant has a nonvalved end plate that is either 185 mm^2 (model M3-185) or 245 mm^2 (model M3-245). They all have different thicknesses and shapes, which may be more important for ease of implantation than outcomes. There are insufficient data on the new Ahmed M4 model, either anecdotally or in the literature, so I will not comment on this implant except to say that the end plate is not flexible and is encased in Medpor (Stryker Corp, Kalamazoo, Michigan). This end-plate material allows surrounding tissue to grow into it, which reportedly results in less diplopia and a minimized hypertensive phase, claims that need to be confirmed in a prospective randomized trial.

Gedde SJ, ed. *Curbside Consultation in Glaucoma:*
49 Clinical Questions, Second Edition (pp 207–209)
© 2015 Taylor & Francis Group

Prospective, randomized trials comparing aqueous shunts have taught us that larger implants likely result in lower intraocular pressure (IOP) in the long term. Comparing the original single- to double-plate Molteno, Heuer et al[2] found that the double-plate implant had a higher success rate at 2 years (71%) compared with the single-plate implant (46%), better percent IOP lowering (46% vs 25%), and less of a hypertensive phase than the single plate. However, there were more serious complications related to the double-plate implant, including suprachoroidal hemorrhage, flat anterior chamber, corneal edema, and phthisis bulbi. There may be an upper limit of benefit of end-plate size, however, as Britt et al[3] subsequently found no differences in outcomes when they compared the Baerveldt 500-mm^2 implant with the 350-mm^2 version in a prospective clinical trial. A retrospective comparison by Seah et al[4] found no difference in final IOP between patients who had the Baerveldt 250-mm^2 vs 350-mm^2 implant. A prospective randomized trial comparing these 2 end-plate sizes is under way. The 3-year results of both the Ahmed Baerveldt Comparison (ABC)[5] and the Ahmed Versus Baerveldt (AVB)[6] Studies showed an approximate 1.5- to 2-mm Hg lower IOP in the Baerveldt 101-350 model group compared with the smaller Ahmed FP7 group, with more serious complications in the larger end-plate Baerveldt group. Similar to the original studies comparing the single- vs. double-plate Molteno implants, there may be a trade-off in terms of larger implants leading to slightly lower IOPs but more complications.

The difference between the valved (Ahmed) and nonvalved (Baerveldt and Molteno) implants seem most relevant for the early postoperative period, but some have hypothesized that the long-term IOP is lower in nonvalved implants because they need to be completely occluded for the first 4 to 6 weeks to prevent severe hypotony-related complications and therefore result in less inflammatory cells and proteins in the bleb postoperatively and ultimately less scarring. The concept of a valve is a good one, although most of us have seen IOPs lower than the advertised opening pressure of 8 mm Hg. I think of the valve as more of a restrictive device. The importance of this is that there is no need to occlude the Ahmed implant's tube because the IOP rarely goes so low as to cause severe hypotony-related complications such as choroidal hemorrhages, retinal detachments, and flat chambers like the nonvalved implants if they are not tied off.[7]

I apply the knowledge generated by clinical trials to my clinical practice by using implants with a larger end plate in patients who need very low IOPs (such as patients with severe glaucoma, normal-tension glaucoma, or progression of glaucoma at normal IOPs) or in those who need low IOP with no or few glaucoma medications. The probability of achieving these outcomes (although rarely in the same patient) seems better with implants that have larger surface areas. Conversely, in patients who have acutely elevated IOP without glaucoma damage but require IOPs in the upper-normal range, such as those with neovascular glaucoma, I am comfortable using the smaller implants since they are easier to implant and offer, in the case of the Ahmed, reliable immediate IOP lowering due to the valve. In addition, the larger implants appear to predispose to chronic hypotony, and this is more likely to occur in patients with systemically caused uveitis; therefore, I use an implant with a smaller end plate in such patients. For the average patients with open-angle glaucoma, all 3 implants generally perform well, and I believe surgeon preference should prevail.

Pediatric patients who require an aqueous shunt present special challenges. The vigorous healing response in children may lead to a very thick, encapsulated bleb and higher IOPs, which I counter by using a larger implant. There have not been clinical trials done in pediatric patients with glaucoma. However, in our own retrospective study, 62 patients younger than 18 years (23 primary and 39 secondary childhood glaucomas) who had Baerveldt implant surgery had surgical success rates of 80% at 1 year, 67% at 2 years, and 60% out to 108 months.[8] This is my preferred operation and implant in pediatric patients who have failed angle surgery or as a primary operation in those who are not good candidates for initial angle surgery.

References

1. Gedde SJ, Panarelli JF, Banitt MR, Lee RK. Evidenced-based comparison of aqueous shunts. Curr Opin Ophthalmol. 2013;24:87-95.
2. Heuer DK, Lloyd MA, Abrams DA, et al. Which is better? One or two? A randomized clinical trial of single-plate versus double-plate Molteno implantation for glaucomas in aphakia and pseudophakia. *Ophthalmology.* 1992;99:1512-1519.
3. Britt MT, LaBree LD, Lloyd MA, et al. Randomized clinical trial of the 350-mm^2 versus the 500-mm^2 Baerveldt implant: longer term results: is bigger better? *Ophthalmology.* 1999;106:2312-2318.
4. Seah SKL, Gazzard G, Aung T. Intermediate-term outcome of Baerveldt glaucoma implants in Asian eyes. *Ophthalmology.* 2003;110:888-894.
5. Barton K, Feuer WJ, Budenz DL, Schiffman J, Costa VP, Godfrey DG, Buys YM; Ahmed Baerveldt Comparison Study Group. Three-year treatment outcomes in the Ahmed Baerveldt Comparison Study. *Ophthalmology.* 2014;121:1547-1557.
6. Christakis PG, Tsai JC, Kalenak JW, et al. The Ahmed versus Baerveldt Study: Three-year treatment outcomes. *Ophthalmology.* 2013;120: 2232-2240.
7. Law SK, Kalenak JW, Connor TB Jr, Pulido JS, Han DP, Mieler WF. Retinal complications after aqueous shunt surgical procedures for glaucoma. *Arch Ophthalmol.* 1996;114:1473-1480.
8. Budenz DL, Gedde SJ, Brandt JD, et al. Baerveldt glaucoma implant in the management of refractory childhood glaucomas. *Ophthalmology.* 2004;111:2204-2210.

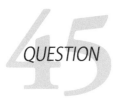

DOES CATARACT EXTRACTION PRODUCE A SIGNIFICANT AND SUSTAINED INTRAOCULAR PRESSURE REDUCTION? WHEN SHOULD I PERFORM A COMBINED PROCEDURE VS CATARACT EXTRACTION ALONE?

Igor Estrovich, MD and
Steven L. Mansberger, MD, MPH

Many retrospective studies have suggested that cataract extraction has an intraocular pressure (IOP) lowering effect in patients with and without glaucoma. The Ocular Hypertension Treatment Study[1] recently evaluated the effect of cataract extraction on IOP in untreated patients with ocular hypertension. The average reduction in IOP was 4 mm Hg or 16.5% postoperatively (Figure 45-1). Approximately 70% of patients had more than 10% IOP lowering, about 19% had no significant change (0% to 9% decrease) in IOP, and about 11% experienced an increase in IOP from baseline (1% to 18% increase). The study found that mean IOP did not return to baseline over 3 years, which suggests long-term IOP reduction (Figure 45-1). Unfortunately, the only predictor of higher IOP response was higher preoperative IOP. For example, the reduction averaged 11% in eyes with IOP between 21 and 22.3 mm Hg before surgery but 22.5% when the preoperative IOP was between 25 and 32 mm Hg. Other factors, including age, sex, race, and central corneal thickness, were not predictive. This information presents a double-edged sword: individuals with higher pressures are more likely to achieve greater pressure reduction, but these same individuals are also at higher risk for glaucoma progression and may require more definitive interventions to control eye pressure in the future.

Other studies in patients with glaucoma have shown similar IOP-lowering results (10% to 20% IOP lowering) with cataract extraction alone. They have also suggested that pseudoexfoliation patients may have more IOP lowering than age- and IOP-matched normal or primary open-angle glaucoma (POAG) eyes; however, pseudoexfoliation is a risk factor for extreme IOP rises in the early postoperative period. Few studies have examined long-term IOP reduction after cataract extraction in other secondary glaucomas such as pigmentary glaucoma and inflammatory glaucoma. The data in these conditions are unclear.

As suggested above, a critical factor to recommending a surgical option is the likelihood of uncontrolled IOP in the early postoperative period that results in significant optic disc damage

Gedde SJ, ed. *Curbside Consultation in Glaucoma:*
49 Clinical Questions, Second Edition (pp 211–214)
© 2015 Taylor & Francis Group

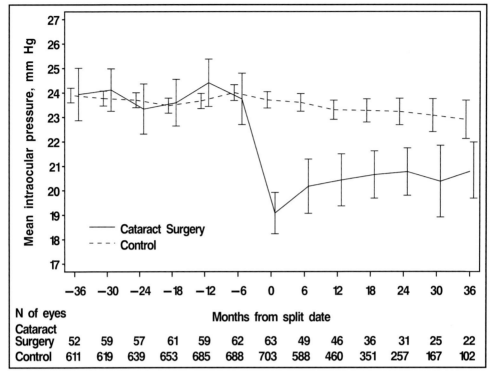

Figure 45-1. Data from the Ocular Hypertensive Treatment Study demonstrate an IOP reduction of 4 mm Hg following phacoemulsification and sustained for 3 years. Reprinted from *Ophthalmology*, 119(9), Mansberger SL, Gordon MO, Jampel H, et al, Reduction in intraocular pressure after cataract extraction: the ocular hypertension study, pp 1826–1831, Copyright 2012, with permission from Elsevier.

and/or visual field loss. Even in normal eyes, approximately 70% of patients may experience IOP elevation to 30 mm Hg or more in the first 12 hours following uncomplicated phacoemulsification.[2] Retained viscoelastic or lens fragments, uncontrolled inflammation, corticosteroid response, or unanticipated surgical complications can extend this period significantly. Thus, even in patients with stable but advanced glaucoma, one must consider whether the optic nerve could tolerate a short-term pressure elevation. Overall, the surgeon should inform cataract surgery patients that they may rarely require emergent glaucoma surgery if their IOP becomes too high in the postoperative period.

Several studies have evaluated the mechanism of IOP lowering with cataract surgery. They can be generally divided into "mechanical" and "biologic" hypotheses. The mechanical hypotheses include (1) increased surface area exposure of trabecular meshwork because of angle widening with cataract surgery and (2) the intraocular lens creating tension in the lens zonule and longitudinal muscle of the ciliary body, which opens the trabecular meshwork spaces (similar to the miotic effect on IOP lowering). In support of these hypotheses, studies suggest that patients with shallow chambers or narrow angles may have a greater amount of IOP lowering after cataract extraction. Ex vivo studies have shown greater facility of outflow with tension on the lens zonule. The biologic hypotheses include activation of proteinases and macrophage activity by phacoemulsification, fluid dynamics during cataract surgery, and/or inflammation. These activities increase the facility of outflow through the conventional and uveoscleral outflow pathways.

Table 45-1 includes the ideal patient characteristics for cataract surgery alone, combined cataract and glaucoma surgery, and glaucoma surgery alone. For glaucoma surgery, we prefer

---

Table 45-1
Surgical Plan Recommendations Based on Patient Characteristics

Surgical Option	*Ideal Patient Characteristics*
Cataract surgery alone	• Stable, early glaucoma on 2 ocular hypotensive medications or less • Able to tolerate an early cataract postoperative IOP elevation • Narrow angles or pseudoexfoliation that may result in greater IOP lowering
Cataract and glaucoma surgery	• Uncontrolled IOP • Inability to tolerate a short-term elevation in IOP from cataract surgery alone • Rapidly progressing glaucoma • Desire to reduce or eliminate ocular hypotensive medications • Need to lower IOP by more than 15% postoperatively
Glaucoma surgery alone	• Poor visual potential despite cataract extraction • High risk of cataract extraction compromising concurrent trabeculectomy

---

trabeculectomy surgery to lower IOP and avoid long-term ocular hypotensive medications, while some surgeons prefer primary seton placement. In situations where the pressure does not need to be lowered so drastically, surgeons may recommend the iStent, trabectome, and other ab interno trabecular bypass surgeries. These emerging therapies forfeit the magnitude of IOP reduction to gain a safer risk profile and shorter postoperative course. These surgeries usually result in IOP in the mid to high teens with ocular hypotensive medications and frequently require subsequent glaucoma surgery.

Finally, one must use a holistic approach. Elderly or systemically sick patients with a modest life expectancy or difficulty returning for postoperative care may elect to forgo glaucoma surgery despite clear progression. Conversely, patients with stable disease but a strong desire to be independent from eye drops may ask to have concurrent glaucoma surgery. In either case, one must engage in an earnest and thorough discussion about the benefits and limitations of each approach to ensure that patient expectations are aligned with the anticipated outcome.

Summary

We recommend cataract extraction alone in patients with glaucoma who are stable on 2 or fewer ocular hypotensive medications, are able to tolerate a postoperative pressure spike, or may have a greater than average response due to a narrow angle (see Table 45-1). Patients who meet these criteria but have a strong desire to be eye drop independent may benefit from glaucoma surgery. Trabeculectomy and cataract extraction should be offered to patients who have uncontrolled IOP and glaucomatous progression, have a low preoperative or target pressure, or are at high risk of losing vision due to a short-term IOP elevation (see Table 45-1). Surgeons should consider glaucoma surgery without cataract surgery if the visual potential is poor or if there is a high risk of cataract extraction compromising concurrent trabeculectomy.

References

1. Mansberger SL, Gordon MO, Jampel H, et al. Reduction in intraocular pressure after cataract extraction: the Ocular Hypertension Treatment Study. *Ophthalmology.* 2012;119(9):1826-1831.
2. Rainer G, Menapace R, Schmid KE, et al. Natural course of intraocular pressure after cataract surgery with sodium chondroitin sulfate 4%-sodium hyaluronate 3% (Viscoat). *Ophthalmology.* 2005;112(10):1714-1718.

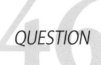

IS CATARACT SURGERY A USEFUL TREATMENT FOR ANGLE CLOSURE GLAUCOMA?

Dennis Lam, MD, FRCOphth; Vineet Ratra, DNB, FRCS(Ed); and Enne Liang, PhD

In the past decade, advances in anterior segment imaging techniques have clearly established the role of the lens in the pathogenesis of primary angle closure glaucoma (PACG). Eyes at increased risk for PACG are small with decreased axial length, shallow anterior chamber depth, and narrow filtration angle width associated with a proportionately large lens.[1] Treatment of a causative factor is preferable and more likely to result in good outcomes. It is here that the role of clear corneal phacoemulsification cataract surgery has become a choice in the treatment of PACG.

Management of patients with angle closure begins with evaluation of the angle to determine the mechanism of angle closure. The primary aim is to get the intraocular pressure (IOP) under control. In cases of acute primary angle closure (APAC), we need to break the acute attack. Laser peripheral iridotomy (LPI) is done to treat pupillary block and equalize the pressure between the anterior and posterior chambers, flatten the iris configuration, and cause a widening of the iridocorneal angle. Alternatively, argon laser peripheral iridoplasty (ALPI) can be used to mechanically pull open the angle and get quick normalization of IOP even in refractory cases when medical therapy has been shown to be ineffective. Anterior chamber paracentesis provides instantaneous relief of symptoms and prevents further optic nerve and trabecular meshwork damage secondary to the acutely raised IOP. It helps in allowing earlier LPI but can be associated with decompression syndrome if the IOP is lowered too suddenly and drastically. Our data have shown good safety and efficacy with these treatments when performed properly.[2,3]

Cataract surgery is the only treatment alternative that corrects the anatomic predisposition responsible for angle closure. It eliminates pupillary block and decreases angle crowding. The reduced iridotrabecular proximity improves aqueous access to the trabecular meshwork. Additional mechanisms described include relieving compression of the trabecular meshwork and the canal of Schlemm by a rearward traction on the anterior ciliary body by the zonules. There is also decreased

Gedde SJ, ed. *Curbside Consultation in Glaucoma:*
49 Clinical Questions, Second Edition (pp 215–217)
© 2015 Taylor & Francis Group

aqueous production from traction on the ciliary body by the zonules in the presence of a contracting capsule.

In a subgroup of patients with mild to moderate glaucomatous optic neuropathy and extensive peripheral anterior synechiae (PAS) of less than 1 year duration, goniosynechialysis (GSL) has an 80% success rate and is most successful with concurrent lens extraction. It involves mechanically stripping PAS away from the trabecular meshwork using a viscoelastic or a cyclodialysis spatula under direct visualization with a Swan Jacob lens. It can, however, be associated with postoperative IOP spikes secondary to retained viscoelastic, hyphema, iris pigment release, and subsequent inflammation.

The role of cataract surgery in PACG has been supported by randomized controlled trials. In patients with APAC, phacoemulsification has been found to be more effective in preventing IOP rise than LPI, after aborting the acute attack, and resulted in a significantly more opened angle compared with LPI.[4] The outflow facility determines the IOP-lowering effect, and long-term IOP reduction is achieved following cataract surgery.

Cataract surgery has also been found to be a useful tool in chronic angle closure glaucoma (CACG). Phacoemulsification is an alternative to trabeculectomy as an initial surgical option in medically uncontrolled CACG eyes without cataract.[5] Phacoemulsification is associated with fewer complications than trabeculectomy with mitomycin-C, but IOP control is better maintained with trabeculectomy. The complications associated with trabeculectomy alone are higher and include cataract formation, overfiltration, wound leak, and failure of the trabeculectomy. In the presence of a clear lens, there is limited literature on the role of combined phacotrabeculectomy.

Surgery in these patients can be fraught with difficulties.[4] In patients with APAC, cataract surgery is ideally undertaken once the inflammation subsides, a month or so after breaking the acute attack and doing an LPI. In the event that the acute attack cannot be broken, one needs to operate early. Surgery in this setting is more difficult, as these eyes are inflamed and painful. It is preferable to do the surgery under a peribulbar block. To deepen the anterior chamber, preoperative hyperosmotic agents can be used to dehydrate the vitreous and/or a vitreous tap can be performed. Several other problems can be encountered in cataract surgery in patients with angle closure. The cornea in these patients may appear cloudy due to reduced endothelial cell counts and may have microcystic changes from elevated IOP. The liberal use of dispersive viscoelastic protects further endothelial cell loss. Floppy iris is common, and the use of preoperative atropine and intraoperative intracameral diluted adrenaline dilates the pupil and restores the iris rigidity. The other surgical principles include adequate preoperative IOP control, gentle decompression, proper wound construction with gentle slow hydrodissection, and low-flow parameters. Small pupils would need either pupil expansion rings or iris retractors. Iris manipulation is associated with more inflammation and postoperative IOP spikes. Postoperative inflammation can be severe with fibrin formation and may necessitate the use of tissue plasminogen activator (TPA). Intraoperative triamcinolone acetate and the use of subconjunctival corticosteroids help reduce inflammation. There is also a higher risk of zonular dialysis, necessitating the need for capsular tension rings. Malignant glaucoma can occur postoperatively. The incidence of postoperative cystoid macular edema is also higher, and topical nonsteroidal anti-inflammatory drugs should be used pre- and postoperatively to reduce the risk. Meticulous planning, anticipation of problems, careful management should problems occur, and an experienced skillful surgeon reduce the risk of complications.

References

1. Tarongoy P, Ho CL, Walton DS. Angle-closure glaucoma: the role of the lens in the pathogenesis, prevention, and treatment. *Surv Ophthalmol.* 2009;54(2):211-225.

2. Lam DS, Chua JK, Tham CC, Lai JS. Efficacy and safety of immediate anterior chamber paracentesis in the treatment of acute primary angle-closure glaucoma: a pilot study. *Ophthalmology.* 2002;109(1):64-70.

3. Ritch R, Tham CC, Lam DS. Argon laser peripheral iridoplasty (ALPI): an update. *Surv Ophthalmol.* 2007;52(3):279-288.

4. Lam DSC, Leung DYL, Tham CCY, et al. Randomized trial of early phacoemulsification versus peripheral iridotomy to prevent intraocular pressure rise after acute primary angle closure. *Ophthalmology.* 2008;115(7):1134-1140.

5. Tham CCY, Kwong YYY, Baig N, Leung DYL, Li FCH, Lam DSC. Phacoemulsification versus trabeculectomy in medically uncontrolled chronic angle-closure glaucoma without cataract. *Ophthalmology.* 2013;120(1):62-67.

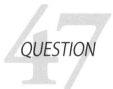

Does the Presence of Glaucoma Influence Your Choice of Intraocular Lens Implant?

Joshua C. Teichman, MD, MPH, FRCSC and
Iqbal Ike K. Ahmed, MD, FRCSC

Presently, a variety of premium intraocular lenses (IOLs) exist, including aspheric IOLs, astigmatism-correcting toric IOLs, diffractive multifocal IOLs, refractive multifocal IOLs, bifocal IOLs, accommodating IOLs, and combinations of these lenses. Moreover, premium IOLs may be available as a 1-piece platform, a 3-piece platform, a plate-haptic platform, or with iris-claw fixation. The surgeon's options for choice of IOL are expanding rapidly.

Currently, there is a paucity of data regarding the use of premium IOLs in patients with glaucoma; hence, the use of premium IOLs in the setting of glaucoma remains controversial.[1] Concerns regarding implanting premium IOLs in patients with glaucoma generally revolve around a few key areas: the decrease in contrast sensitivity attributable to glaucoma and many multifocal IOLs; the increased risk of postoperative capsular contraction syndrome with lack of zonular support in patients with glaucoma, specifically those with pseudoexfoliation syndrome; future difficulties in monitoring glaucoma progression; issues with preoperative measurements in glaucomatous eyes, including artifacts caused by hypotony or intraocular hypertension; bleb-induced astigmatism; and ocular surface disease degrading visual quality.

The visual field changes in patients with glaucoma are well known. A recent study looking specifically at the change in visual field after implantation of a multifocal IOL revealed a decrease in mean deviation using the size III protocol and a decrease in mean sensitivity using the size V protocol compared with phakic controls.[2] However, this study was not performed in patients with glaucoma specifically. Another consideration with regard to monitoring patients with multifocal IOLs is their effect on retinal nerve fiber layer imaging. One study revealed that multifocal IOLs may cause wavy artifacts on optical coherence tomography images.[3]

A reduction in contrast sensitivity, specifically at mesopic levels, is correlated with visual field loss in patients with glaucoma.[4] The introduction of aspheric IOLs that induce negative spherical aberration has afforded surgeons another option for managing cataracts in patients with glaucoma.

Gedde SJ, ed. *Curbside Consultation in Glaucoma:*
49 Clinical Questions, Second Edition (pp 219–221)
© 2015 Taylor & Francis Group

These lenses may decrease glare, haloes, and other unwanted visual phenomena attributable to spherical aberration. As patients with glaucoma already have decreased contrast sensitivity and increased glare-like phenomena, these lenses may ameliorate some of this loss by controlling for the spherical aberration induced by the cornea. It is important to mention, however, that patients with glaucoma may have weak zonules, especially those with pseudoexfoliation syndrome. These patients may be predisposed to IOL decentration. The decentration of aspheric IOLs may induce further higher order aberrations. In patients in whom zonular stability may be an issue, a 3-piece IOL placed in the capsular bag may be a better long-term option.

Multifocal IOLs have multiple focal distances, and in patients who have had them implanted, as few as 20% require glasses for near. However, there is a trade-off. These patients often experience unwanted glare and haloes and may have reduced contrast sensitivity. Because both glaucoma and multifocal IOLs decrease contrast sensitivity, there has been significant debate over whether it is appropriate to implant a multifocal IOL into an eye with glaucomatous damage. At the present time, the only study assessing multifocal IOLs in patients with eye disease was performed by Kamath et al[5] and published in 2000. Kamath et al studied 133 eyes, 29 of which had glaucoma or ocular hypertension. Eleven eyes with glaucoma and 6 with ocular hypertension received a multifocal IOL, and 12 received a monofocal IOL. The study revealed that the only difference in outcomes was that the multifocal IOL group had better near visual acuity. This is a small sample size, but it may demonstrate that patients with glaucoma may benefit from multifocal IOLs. Moreover, some of the issues with decreased contrast sensitivity may be improved with the newer aspheric multifocal IOLs presently available.

In patients with previous filtration surgery, the 2 major concerns are preoperative measurement accuracy and preexisting astigmatism. With regard to measurements, the use of noncontact biometry is encouraged in softer eyes, so as to not compress the globe, creating artifact. In patients presenting for phacotrabeculectomy, a decrease in axial length ranging from 0.1 to 0.9 mm has been observed, and aiming for slight myopia may reduce hyperopic surprises. In eyes with a filtering bleb, there may be significant with-the-rule astigmatism, and if stable, one should consider the use of a toric IOL. Again, the issue of zonular weakness is important to assess preoperatively and intraoperatively. Rotation of a toric IOL may potentially decrease its efficacy or, even worse, produce further astigmatism.

The question often becomes which lens to implant in patients with pseudoexfoliation syndrome. We find that this is usually a question of severity. In those with significant zonular weakness and nondilating pupils, it may be a challenge to merely extract the lens safely, often with the help of iris hooks or pupil expansion rings, as well as capsular tension rings or segments. These patients may require a 3-piece IOL sutured to the iris or sclera, or an iris-claw lens. For these patients, a spherical IOL may be the safest bet, although certainly toric and multifocal IOLs have been used if optimal centration can be achieved.

On the other end of the spectrum, in patients who dilate well, have good capsular support, and are ocular hypertensives or have mild stable glaucomatous changes, then almost all of the aforementioned premium IOLs may be a reasonable option.

Glaucoma is a spectrum of disease, from those who were incidentally found to have elevated intraocular pressures and trace changes on optical coherence tomography (OCT) to those who are bilaterally blind. Although it is obvious that the latter group would not benefit from the advanced optics of a premium IOL, it is also not fair to label all patients with glaucoma as ineligible, as many of the former may receive benefit and improved quality of life from these lenses.

References

1. Kumar BV, Phillips RP, Prasad S. Multifocal intraocular lenses in the setting of glaucoma. *Curr Opin Ophthalmol.* 2007;18(1):62-66.
2. Aychoua N, Montolio FGJ, Jansonius NM. Influence of multifocal intraocular lenses on standard automated perimetry test results. *JAMA Ophthalmol.* 2013;131(4):481-485.
3. Inoue M, Bissen-Miyajima H, Yoshino M, Suzuki T. Wavy horizontal artifacts on optical coherence tomography line-scanning images caused by diffractive multifocal intraocular lenses. *J Cataract Refract Surg.* 2009;35(7):1239-1243.
4. Hawkins AS, Szlyk JP, Ardickas Z, Alexander KR, Wilensky JT. Comparison of contrast sensitivity, visual acuity, and Humphrey visual field testing in patients with glaucoma. *J Glaucoma.* 2003;12(2):134-138.
5. Kamath GG, Prasad S, Danson A, Phillips RP. Visual outcome with the array multifocal intraocular lens in patients with concurrent eye disease. *J Cataract Refract Surg.* 2000;26(4):576-581.

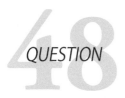

IN WHICH GLAUCOMA PATIENTS SHOULD I CONSIDER CYCLODESTRUCTION?

Malik Y. Kahook, MD; Jeffrey R. SooHoo, MD;
and Leonard K. Seibold, MD

Cycloablative procedures target the ciliary body epithelium, which produces aqueous humor, to reduce intraocular pressure (IOP). Various methods of cyclodestruction, including diathermy, ultrasonic energy, and cryotherapy, have existed for many years and were traditionally reserved for end-stage glaucoma. Newer cyclodestructive procedures soon replaced these earlier methods, beginning with Xenon arc photocoagulation and later followed by Nd:YAG and diode laser photocoagulation. Currently, the diode laser is the most widely used for cyclophotocoagulation (CPC), and treatment can be delivered by either the transscleral route with a G-probe (Figure 48-1) or by the endoscopic route.

We often use transscleral CPC for patients with advanced glaucoma and poor IOP control, despite maximal medical therapy, who have also failed one or two incisional surgeries. Other potential candidates include patients with aphakic glaucoma, neovascular glaucoma (NVG), and glaucoma after penetrating keratoplasty. These patients are at an increased risk for complications or frank failure and may benefit from CPC as first-line surgical therapy when medications fail to control IOP. Eyes with no light perception vision, pain, and high IOP also benefit from this noninvasive procedure. Recent reports indicate that transscleral CPC may be an appropriate first-line option in patients who experience difficulty with follow-up or in populations with limited resources for medical or surgical therapy.[1]

The most common complications of transscleral CPC include pain, inflammation, large fluctuations of IOP, and hyphema. These complications remain a major obstacle to more prevalent use of CPC. Other less common complications of transscleral diode therapy include conjunctival burns, cataract formation, irregular/tonic pupil, and cystoid macular edema.

Intraocular pressure spikes after CPC can usually be controlled with topical medical therapy. Contreras and colleagues[2] reported that 10.8% of eyes treated with CPC experienced an IOP

Gedde SJ, ed. *Curbside Consultation in Glaucoma:*
49 Clinical Questions, Second Edition (pp 223–226)
© 2015 Taylor & Francis Group

Figure 48-1. The G-probe is used with transscleral CPC. The quartz tip indents the conjunctiva and directs the laser energy through the sclera to the ciliary body.

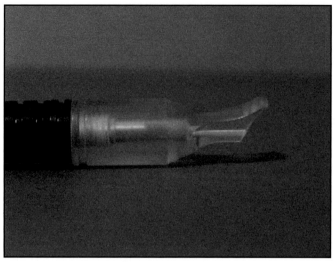

spike. While elevations in IOP may be seen with all forms of glaucoma, patients with NVG are more prone to this complication and should be watched closely. We see patients on the first postoperative day and institute topical and/or oral therapy to control IOP spikes if they occur. In most cases, the pressure is lowered and a slow wean off of medical therapy is possible.

Postoperative hypotony after CPC is a dreaded complication that often requires intense therapy and close follow-up to lessen the chance of long-term morbidity. Our usual treatment regimen consists of both long-term topical corticosteroids and cycloplegics after eliminating other possible causes of hypotony such as retinal detachment and/or choroidal detachments. Despite close follow-up and treatment, eyes with chronic hypotony will have decreased vision and may become phthisical and/or require enucleation. The best way to avoid complications from hypotony is to prevent its occurrence in the first place. The laser is initially set to 2000 mW and a duration of 2000 ms; the power is increased in increments of 250 mW until the first audible "pop" is heard. Following this, we decrease the power by 250 mW and proceed with treatment. We do not perform 360 degrees of CPC in any of our patients. We typically start by treating 270 degrees and observe closely. If IOP lowering is insufficient, the remaining 90 degrees can be treated in a second session. This method helps prevent a dramatic drop in pressure that may be irreversible, especially in patients with NVG who tend to experience more post-CPC hypotony compared with other groups. Another option is to use the "slow-burn" technique, which requires the surgeon to apply a lower power (1250 mW) but for a longer duration (4000 ms). Regardless of what parameters are used, an average of 4 to 6 spots can be placed in each quadrant for a total treatment between 20 and 24 applications.

Vision loss after CPC is the most feared posttreatment complication. While well known, there are few data as to the true incidence and etiology of vision loss after cycloablation. Some factors leading to vision loss include development of cataract, high or low IOP, chronic uveitis, and cystoid macular edema, among others. Many of the complications linked to transscleral diode therapy result from the transmission of energy across the sclera to tissue adjacent to the ciliary body or from the excessive energy application required to treat the targeted tissue.

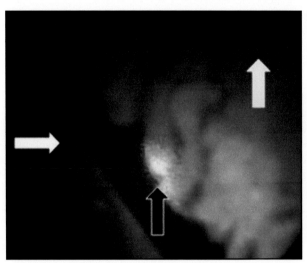

Figure 48-2. Endoscopic view during endocyclophotocoagulation showing ciliary processes (black arrow), iris (yellow arrow), and anterior capsule (white arrow).

Endocyclophotocoagulation

Endoscopic cyclophotocoagulation (ECP) is a method of cycloablation performed with an 810-nm diode laser, a 175-W Xenon light source, and a helium-neon laser aiming beam combined into a single intraocular probe (Endo Optiks, Little Silver, New Jersey). The endoscopic imaging system allows for direct visualization of ciliary processes during treatment, resulting in a more precise and titratable treatment (Figure 48-2). The power is set at 0.25 W on continuous mode, with tissue whitening and shrinkage of the ciliary processes as the goal of treatment. Collateral tissue damage is limited in experienced hands, thus decreasing the potential for postoperative complications.

The efficacy of ECP for the treatment of refractory glaucoma has been reported by Chen and coworkers[3] in 68 eyes of 68 patients. They noted a mean decrease in IOP of 34% with an average follow-up of 12.9 months. Treatment complications included anterior chamber fibrin, hyphema, cystoid macular edema, and choroidal effusion. No cases of hypotony or phthisis were observed. Other studies have also shown safe and successful outcomes from ECP treatment comparable to both glaucoma drainage device implantation and trabeculectomy.[4,5]

Appropriate patient selection is the key to successful outcomes with ECP. In the past, we performed ECP at earlier stages of glaucoma when combined with cataract extraction. Our continued experience with this approach and constant monitoring of our results has revealed that many of these patients required reinitiation of their medications after 12 to 18 months of follow-up. This has led us to a change in patient selection toward those with more advanced disease and in those whose options might be more limited in the setting of uncontrolled IOP and advancing glaucomatous optic neuropathy. We now reserve ECP for patients with glaucoma in 3 specific categories. The first category includes patients undergoing phacoemulsification who have had a history of poor adherence to prescribed topical medications or those with observed intolerance to medical therapy. The goal in these patients is to achieve IOP control without reliance on medical therapy. Patients with poorly controlled glaucoma despite maximal medical therapy in the setting of failed previous filtration or glaucoma drainage device surgery and limited healthy conjunctiva make up the second group. The goal in this category is to achieve improved pressure control in patients who previously would have undergone transscleral CPC. Success can be achieved without the collateral tissue damage that occurs with CPC.[6] The third group is made up of patients who have marginal IOP control after glaucoma drainage device surgery and require further IOP lowering.[7] These patients tend to do well with combined cataract + ECP or ECP alone and may reach goal IOP synergistically with a functioning drainage device in place. Due to limited visualization and potential damage to the crystalline lens, ECP should be performed only in aphakic eyes, pseudophakic eyes, or in conjunction with cataract surgery.

Few prospective studies have reported on the utility of ECP in decreasing IOP or its effect on decreasing dependence on topical medications.[8] We have found that treating 360 degrees through 2 clear cornea incisions results in improved IOP lowering that can be long lasting without an increase in inflammation or hypotony. The second incision, constructed 100 to 120 degrees away from the first, allows for the treatment of tissue underneath the initial clear cornea incision. We have witnessed an average IOP decrease of ~30% when treating 360 degrees through a clear cornea incision approach. In our experience, 60% of patients are able to decrease the use of topical medications postoperatively. There have been no cases of chronic hypotony or phthisis in our experience to date.

Conclusion

Cycloablative procedures have played an important role in treating glaucomas refractory to other methods of IOP control. While transscleral CPC has often been reserved for patients with poor vision, careful titration of laser spot application and energy used can allow for both safe and effective treatment in patients with functional vision. ECP is a method of cycloablation that allows for direct visualization of targeted tissue and has found a role in treating specific categories of patients with glaucoma in our practice. More prospective research is needed to better understand the differences between CPC and ECP as well as their role in treating glaucoma in different patient populations.

References

1. Lai JS, Tham CC, Chan JC, Lam DS. Diode laser transscleral cyclophotocoagulation as primary surgical treatment for medically uncontrolled chronic angle closure glaucoma: long-term clinical outcomes. *J Glaucoma.* 2005;14(2):114-119.
2. Contreras I, Noval S, Gonzalez Martin-Moro J, Rebolleda G, Munoz-Negrete FJ. IOP spikes following contact transscleral diode laser cyclophotocoagulation. *Arch Soc Esp Oftalmol.* 2004;79(3):105-109.
3. Chen J, Cohn RA, Lin SC, et al. Endoscopic photocoagulation of the ciliary body for treatment of refractory glaucomas. *Am J Ophthalmol.* 1997;124:787.
4. Lima FE, Magacho L, Carvalho DM, Susanna R Jr, Avila MP. A prospective, comparative study between endoscopic cyclophotocoagulation and the Ahmed drainage implant in refractory glaucoma. *J Glaucoma.* 2004;13:233-237.
5. Gayton JL, Van Der Karr M, Sanders V. Combined cataract and glaucoma surgery: trabeculectomy versus endoscopic laser cycloablation. *J Cataract Refract Surg.* 1999;25:1214-1219.
6. Pantcheva MB, Kahook MY, Schuman JS, Noecker RJ. Comparison of acute structural and histopathological changes in human autopsy eyes after endoscopic cyclophotocoagulation and trans-scleral cyclophotocoagulation. *Br J Ophthalmol.* 2007;91(2):248-252.
7. Francis BA, Kawji AS, Vo NT, Dustin L, Chopra V. Endoscopic cyclophotocoagulation (ECP) in the management of uncontrolled glaucoma with prior aqueous tube shunt. *J Glaucoma.* 2011;20(8):523-527.
8. Berke SJ, Sturm RT, Caronia RM, et al. Phacoemulsification combined with endoscopic cyclophotocoagulation in the management of cataract and glaucoma. Paper presented at: The AAO Annual Meeting; November 14, 2006; Las Vegas, NV.

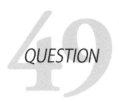

WHAT ARE MIGS?
WHEN SHOULD I USE THEM?

Hady Saheb, MD and
Dima Kalache, MD, CM

The definition of the term *MIGS*, for micro- (or minimally) invasive glaucoma surgery, has varied over time. This definition allows the framing of this category of glaucoma procedures, the optimization of its indications, and the comparison of the efficacy of procedures that share similar features. Microinvasiveness goes beyond the incision size of these procedures. The term *microinvasive* refers to a group of procedures that minimize the level of invasiveness and share a number of common features without minimizing the complexity of the skills required to perform and develop this kind of surgery. Although many of these procedures can be minimally invasive, that is not necessarily the case for all procedures. Hence, *microinvasive* is becoming a more preferred term when describing these newer surgical techniques.

MIGS refers to a group of surgical procedures that share a few preferable qualities.[1] The first is its conjunctival-sparing ab interno microincisional approach. This approach allows for more invasive ab externo surgical procedures if necessary without compromising its successful outcome.[2] Ab interno surgery is performed through a clear corneal incision, sparing the conjunctiva of surgical manipulation and scarring. This approach allows a direct view of anatomic landmarks, which facilitates implantation of incisions or devices within the angle and is easily combined with cataract surgery. The microincision contributes to the intraoperative maintenance of the anterior chamber, minimizes disruption of ocular anatomy and changes in postoperative refractive outcome, and adds to the safety of the procedure. A second feature is a procedure that imposes minimal trauma to the target tissues. An atraumatic approach minimizes inflammation, accelerates postoperative recovery, and maintains anatomy and physiologic outflow pathways. The maintenance of such pathways allows the episcleral venous pressure to provide a natural posttrabecular meshwork outflow resistance to prevent hypotony-related complications. A third feature is the procedure's efficacy, which needs to be at least modest. The fourth feature of MIGS is an extremely high safety profile. These procedures must avoid visually threatening complications seen with other ab externo

Gedde SJ, ed. *Curbside Consultation in Glaucoma:*
49 Clinical Questions, Second Edition (pp 227–230)
© 2015 Taylor & Francis Group

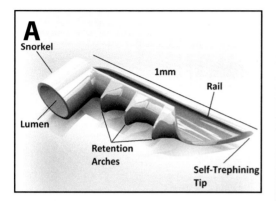

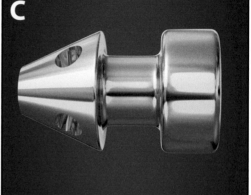

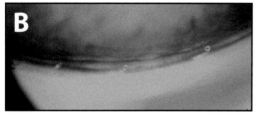

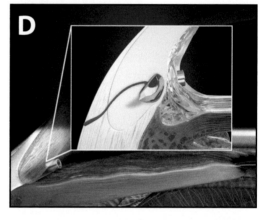

Figure 49-1. (A) iStent trabecular micro-bypass stent. (B) Goniosopic image showing correct placement of 3 iStents through the trabecular meshwork. (C) Second-generation iStent *inject*. (D) Schematic cross-section of angle showing correct placement of iStent *inject*. (E) Istent injector. (Figures A, C, D, E reprinted with permission from Glaukos Corporation. Figure B reprinted with permission of Dr. Ike Ahmed.)

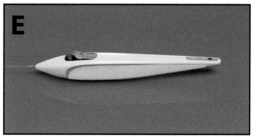

glaucoma surgeries, including hypotony, choroidal effusions, suprachoroidal hemorrhage, anterior chamber shallowing, corneal decompensation, cataract formation, diplopia, and bleb-related complications such as bleb dysesthesia and endophthalmitis. The fifth feature is a rapid recovery for the patient with minimal impact on quality of life.

The iStent (Glaukos Corporation, Laguna Hills, California) is manufactured from heparin-coated titanium in a single-piece design (Figure 49-1). The iStent was best studied in a randomized multicenter clinical trial comparing phacoemulsification with one iStent to phacoemulsification alone in patients with mild to moderate open-angle glaucoma. This study showed a sustained reduction in intraocular pressure (IOP) in both groups, a higher proportion of unmedicated patients with an IOP less than or equal to 21 mm Hg in the iStent group, and a difference in mean IOP between the 2 groups of 1 mm Hg at 24 months. Consistent with the MIGS safety profile, there were no significant differences in adverse events between the 2 groups.[3] Other smaller studies have

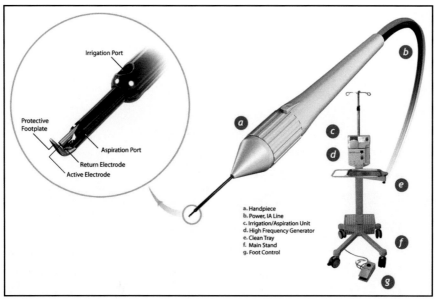

Figure 49-2. Ab interno trabeculotomy Trabectome. (Reprinted with permission of Neomedix Inc.)

supported the role of iStent surgery in patients with pseudoexfoliation and pigmentary glaucoma and the benefit of multiple iStents. The Trabectome (Neomedix, Inc, Tustin, California) removes a strip of trabecular meshwork and inner wall of Schlemm's canal using high-frequency electrocautery (Figure 49-2). The 19.5-gauge handpiece incorporates an insulated footplate that enters Schlemm's canal through the trabecular meshwork. Trabectome results have been reported in an extensive case series showing a reduction in IOP from 24 to 16 mm Hg with a significant reduction in medications, with a slightly increased efficacy in Trabectome-only cases compared with phaco-Trabectome.[4]

Other MIGS options exist, such as Excimer laser trabeculostomy and investigational devices such as the iStent *inject* and the iStent *supra* (Glaukos Corporation; Figure 49-1), Xen Gel Stent (AqueSys, Irvine, California), Hydrus Intracanalicular Implant (Ivantis, Irvine, California), and the CyPass Micro-Stent (Transcend Medical, Menlo Park, California; Figure 49-3).

As the studies have shown modest reductions in IOP, currently MIGS is most suitable for patients with mild to moderate glaucoma damage, ocular hypertension, and modest targeted IOP reductions. These patients also tend to have less diseased physiologic outflow pathways. The ideal timing of MIGS continues to be clarified. Given its efficacy and extremely high safety profile, MIGS can be considered earlier in the glaucoma treatment algorithm than more invasive glaucoma surgeries. Combining MIGS with cataract surgery is currently the most classic indication as risks of an intraocular procedure are already accepted, and this combined surgery has been best studied. Indications for MIGS in the absence of cataract surgery—"solo" MIGS—remain to be determined as appropriate quantification of effect is not yet available in the literature.

We are in an exciting time for glaucoma surgery and MIGS. MIGS is bridging the gap of efficacy and safety between noninvasive options such as medications and laser therapy and the more invasive glaucoma surgeries such as trabeculectomy and glaucoma drainage devices. MIGS may also play a role in medication independence and quality-of-life issues related to medication side effects. We believe important questions remain to be answered regarding the role and indications of MIGS without phacoemulsification, comparative studies between devices, long-term biocompatibility and safety of these devices, and the ability to target implantation of MIGS devices in

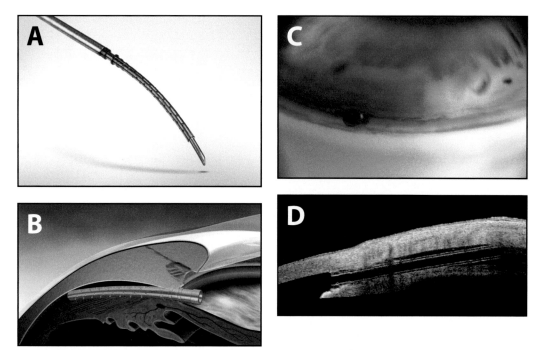

Figure 49-3. (A) Ab interno suprachoroidal CyPass micro-stent. (B) Schematic cross-section showing optimal placement of CyPass micro-stent into suprachoroidal space. (C) Gonioscopic image showing placement of CyPass micro-stent. (D) Visante OCT image showing placement of CyPass micro-stent within suprachoroidal space with surrounding hyporeflectivity representing fluid. (Figures A and B reprinted with permission from Transcend Medical. Figures C and D reprinted with permission from Dr. Ike Ahmed.)

higher outflow areas of the angle. Further evidence and quantification of effect will determine its role in the evolving glaucoma treatment algorithm.

Acknowledgments

I would like to acknowledge Ike Ahmed, who coined the term *MIGS* and played a critical role in the way I think about MIGS, and the late Francisco Fantes for introducing me to MIGS modalities during my fellowship.

References

1. Saheb H, Ahmed IIK. Micro-invasive glaucoma surgery: current perspectives and future directions. *Curr Opin Ophthalmol.* 2012;23(2):96-104.
2. Jea SY, Mosaed S, Vold SD, Rhee DJ. Effect of a failed trabectome on subsequent trabeculectomy. *J Glaucoma.* 2012;21(2):71-75.
3. Craven ER, Katz LJ, Wells JM, Giamporcaro JE; iStent Study Group. Cataract surgery with trabecular micro-bypass stent implantation in patients with mild-to-moderate open-angle glaucoma and cataract: two-year follow-up. *J Cataract Refract Surg.* 2012;38(8):1339-1345.
4. Minckler D, Mosaed S, Dustin L, Ms BF; Trabectome Study Group. Trabectome (trabeculectomy-internal approach): additional experience and extended follow-up. *Trans Am Ophthalmol Soc.* 2008;106:149-160.

FINANCIAL DISCLOSURES

Dr. Iqbal Ike K. Ahmed has interests in Alcon and AMO.

Dr. R. Rand Allingham has no financial or proprietary interest in the materials presented herein.

Dr. Douglas R. Anderson is a consultant for Carl Zeiss Meditec, Inc.

Dr. Husam Ansari receives speakers fees from Alcon and Allergan and consulting fees from Alcon, and Allergan. He receives research support from Allergan and Ivantis.

Dr. Ahmad A. Aref has no financial or proprietary interest in the materials presented herein.

Dr. Michael Banitt has no financial or proprietary interest in the materials presented herein.

Dr. Andrew J. Barkmeier has no financial or proprietary interest in the materials presented herein.

Dr. Keith Barton receives lecture honoraria from Allergan and Pfizer.
He is on the advisory boards of Glaukos, Alcon, Merck, Kowa, Amakem, Thea, Alimera, Refocus, and Ivantis. He is a consultant for Alcon, Aquesys, Ivantis, Refocus, and Carl Zeiss Meditec.
He has received educational grants and research funding from AMO, New World Medical, Alcon, Merck, Allergan, and Refocus. He has stock in AqueSys, Ophthalmic Implants (PTE) Ltd, Vision Futures (UK) and Ltd (director). He has patents for Ophthalmic Implants (PTE) and for Ltd a patent pending.

Dr. Dana M. Blumberg has no financial or proprietary interest in the materials presented herein.

Dr. James D. Brandt is a consultant for Ametek, the manufacturer of both the Ocular Response Analyzer (ORA) and the pneumatonometer.

Dr. Adam C. Breunig has no financial or proprietary interest in the materials presented herein.

Dr. Donald L. Budenz has no financial or proprietary interest in the materials presented herein.

Dr. Joseph Caprioli has no financial or proprietary interest in the materials presented herein.

Dr. Ta Chen Peter Chang has no financial or proprietary interest in the materials presented herein.

Dr. Philip P. Chen has no financial or proprietary interest in the materials presented herein.

Dr. E. Randy Craven has no financial or proprietary interest in the materials presented herein.

Dr. David L. Cute has no financial or proprietary interest in the materials presented herein.

Dr. Igor Estrovich has no financial or proprietary interest in the materials presented herein.

Dr. Ronald L. Fellman has no financial or proprietary interest in the materials presented herein.

Dr. John H. Fingert has no financial or proprietary interest in the materials presented herein.

Dr. David Fleischman has no financial or proprietary interest in the materials presented herein.

Dr. Brian A. Francis has been a paid speaker for Lumenis, Inc. He has received an unrestricted educational research grant from Lumenis.

Dr. Steven J. Gedde has no financial or proprietary interest in the materials presented herein.

Dr. David S. Greenfield has no financial or proprietary interest in the materials presented herein.

Dr. Davinder S. Grover has no financial or proprietary interest in the materials presented herein.

Dr. Gregg A. Heatley has no financial or proprietary interest in the materials presented herein.

Dr. Dale K. Heuer has interests in Aeon Astron (DSMB member) and Innovia (DSMB member).

Dr. Wendy W. Huang has no financial or proprietary interest in the materials presented herein.

Dr. Annisa L. Jamil has no financial or proprietary interest in the materials presented herein.

Dr. Anna K. Junk has no financial or proprietary interest in the materials presented herein.

Dr. Malik Y. Kahook has no financial or proprietary interest in the materials presented herein.

Dr. Dima Kalache has no financial or proprietary interest in the materials presented herein.

Dr. Anne Ko has no financial or proprietary interest in the materials presented herein.

Dr. Dennis Lam has no financial or proprietary interest in the materials presented herein.

Dr. Paul Lee has no financial or proprietary interest in the materials presented herein.

Dr. Richard K. Lee has no financial or proprietary interest in the materials presented herein.

Dr. Christopher Leung has research support from Carl Zeiss Meditec, Optovue, and Tomey, and speaker honorarium for Carl Zeiss Meditec, Tomey, and Global Vision.

Dr. Richard A. Lewis is a consultant for Aerie, Allegan, Alcon, Aquesys, AVS, Envisia, Glaukos, Ivantis, Oculeve, PolyActiva, and ViSci.

Dr. Enne Liang has no financial or proprietary interest in the materials presented herein.

Dr. Jeffrey M. Liebmann has no financial or proprietary interest in the materials presented herein.

Dr. John T. Lind is on the advisory board of Allergan.

Dr. Jane Loman has no financial or proprietary interest in the materials presented herein.

Dr. Steven L. Mansberger is a consultant for Envisia, Welch-Allyn, Allergan, Alcon, Valeant, and Santen. He does research for Allergan, Merck, National Eye Institute, and Mobius.

Dr. Rashmi G. Mathew has no financial or proprietary interest in the materials presented herein.

Dr. Hylton R. Mayer is a speaker and consultant for Bausch and Lomb, Alcon, and Allergan.

Dr. Felipe A. Medeiros has no financial or proprietary interest in the materials presented herein.

Dr. Richard P. Mills has no financial or proprietary interest in the materials presented herein.

Dr. Silvia Orengo-Nania has no financial or proprietary interest in the materials presented herein.

Dr. Joseph F. Panarelli receives lecture fees from Tissue Banks International.

Dr. Sung Chul Park has no financial or proprietary interest in the materials presented herein.

Dr. Richard K. Parrish II is a consultant for Alcon Laboratories, Inc. He is a member of the scientific advisory committee with stock options for Alimera Sciences, Inc. Dr. Parrish is a member of the scientific advisory board with stock options for Aerie Pharmaceuticals, Inc. He has stock options for AqueSys, Inc., and Glaukos Corporation. He is a member of the scientific advisory board with stock options for InnFocus Inc.

Dr. Jody R. Piltz-Seymour has no financial or proprietary interest in the materials presented herein.

Dr. Pradeep Ramulu has research funding from the National Eye Institute and Research to Prevent Blindness and speakers fees from Carl Zeiss Meditec and Tissue Banks International.

Dr. Vineet Ratra has no financial or proprietary interest in the materials presented herein.

Dr. Robert Ritch has no financial or proprietary interest in the materials presented herein.

Dr. Alan L. Robin has financial interests and relationship to Aerie Pharmaceuticals, Allergan, Glaukos Corporation, Merck and Company, Ohr Pharmaceuticals, Sucampo, XLVision, and TEVA Pharmaceuticals.

Dr. Hady Saheb received travel funding from Glaukos, Ivantis and Transcend Medical. He received a research grant from Ivantis. Dr. Saheb is a consultant for Alcon and Allergan.

Dr. Leonard K. Seibold has no financial or proprietary interest in the materials presented herein.

Dr. Bhavna P. Sheth has no financial or proprietary interest in the materials presented herein.

Dr. Paul A. Sidoti receives lecture fees from NeoMedix, Inc.

Dr. Kuldev Singh has interests in Alcon, Allergan, Bausch and Lomb, Santen, Sucampo, and Zeiss.

Dr. Arthur J. Sit is a consultant for AcuMEMS, Inc., Allergan, Inc., and Sensimed AG. He has received research funding from Glaukos Corporation.

Dr. Alon Skaat has no financial or proprietary interest in the materials presented herein.

Dr. Jeffrey R. SooHoo has no financial or proprietary interest in the materials presented herein.

Dr. Angelo P. Tanna has no financial or proprietary interest in the materials presented herein.

Dr. Joshua C. Teichman has no financial or proprietary interest in the materials presented herein.

Dr. Celso Tello has no financial or proprietary interest in the materials presented herein.

Dr. James C. Tsai serves as consultant for Aerie Pharmaceuticals and Amakem.

Dr. Reena S. Vaswani has no financial or proprietary interest in the materials presented herein.

Dr. Martin Wand has no financial or proprietary interest in the materials presented herein.

Dr. Sarah R. Wellik has no financial or proprietary interest in the materials presented herein.

Dr. Darrell WuDunn has no financial or proprietary interest in the materials presented herein.

INDEX

Printed in the United States
by Baker & Taylor Publisher Services